UNDERSTANDING
BACK TROUBLE

UNDERSTANDING
BACK TROUBLE

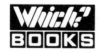

Published by Consumers' Association
and Hodder & Stoughton

Which? Books are commissioned and researched by
The Association for Consumer Research and published by
Consumers' Association, 2 Marylebone Road, NW1 4DX and
Hodder & Stoughton, 47 Bedford Square, London WC1B 3DP

Copyright © 1991 Consumers' Associated Limited
First edition June 1988
Reprinted November 1988
Revised edition March 1991

British Library Cataloguing in Publication Data
Understanding back trouble.
  1. Man. Back. Backache
  I. Consumers' Association
  616.73

ISBN 0 340 55003 1

Originally edited by Edith Rudinger
New research by Janet Pidcock
Cover design by Ivor Claydon
Designed by Paul Saunders
Cover photographs courtesy of the Image Bank/Larry Dale Gordon,
Sally and Richard Greenhill and ACE Photo Agency/Roger Howard

Photoset by Paston Press, Loddon, Norfolk
Printed and bound in Great Britain by Billings
Bookplan Ltd., Worcester

CONTENTS

Contents

Throughout this book for 'he' read 'he or she'

CHAPTER 1

BACKGROUND

BACK pain is a common scourge of humanity – at least in developed countries. There can be few westerners who do not experience it, if only for a short while, at some time in their lives. There is no telling when it will strike, because it need not be preceded by injury: it may be brought on by moderate physical exertion, poor or abnormal posture – or by nothing one can put one's finger on.

No one can ignore back pain when it does strike – usually in the lower back, but it can be anywhere along the length of the spine. It can manifest itself as a 'crick' in the neck, a sharp pain between the shoulder blades, a cramp in the back of the waist, a deep ache across the hips or the arms and legs. Often it can make it difficult, even impossible, to maintain some or all of the commonest human postures – sitting, standing, lying down. It can vary from a feeling of discomfort to one of the most intense kinds of pain known; it can mean a few days off work – or even, very occasionally, prolonged disablement.

Back pain, it goes without saying, is not an illness, but a symptom. It indicates a malfunction of the spine or its supporting musculature, but says nothing about causes; muscle strain, a trapped nerve, spondylitis are just three of the many possible ones. Not all back pain derives from the spine: the symptoms may have quite a different cause, such as gynaecological problems or some type of kidney disease.

Even though most backache is a passing problem, early episodes of back pain should not be ignored. The first two or three episodes may last a few hours, days or weeks, and while they last, the sufferer can usually think of nothing else. But once they are over, they are readily forgotten. Most people, in fact, recover quite quickly, even without treatment. However, these attacks tend to recur; there may be a pattern, perhaps with each successive one lasting longer; eventually the pain may come to stay. It may therefore be wise to establish the cause of even moderate attacks of back pain, in the hope of preventing recurrences.

There are some types of damage stemming from an inherited weakness that cannot be prevented. Some attacks of back pain strike out of the blue, seemingly without any unusual stress or strain, but may nevertheless be the culmination of years of unwitting misuse or of minor incidents in which small aches and pains are disregarded. Some aerobics enthusiasts exercise through sensations of soreness, perhaps 'going for the burn' (that is, deliberately exercising till it hurts). It is not easy to know why some people who do these things are afflicted, and others spared. There may well be a hereditary factor, endowing some people with a tendency to weakness in some of their structures. Very tall people seem to be more at risk than others; also those who are too stout. However, just as some people worry compulsively, yet do not suffer from stomach ulcers, or smoke heavily without getting lung cancer, so there are people who court disaster by lifting heavy weights awkwardly, stooping over their work, sitting slumped in badly designed seating, being overweight – yet are never bothered by back or neck pain.

Nothing to show for it

Sufferers may have the additional problem of convincing others that they are really suffering. The cause of their complaint is not obvious, there is no visible abnormality and there is no objective way of verifying it. When a bone is broken and the limb is put in plaster, everyone knows why you are housebound for a while. With bronchitis and a course of antibiotics, people will accept that you are really ill. But if you have back or neck pain, while everyone will agree that you may need a few days to rest, that may be all. Employers are sometimes intolerant of lost work time (over fifty million working days a year are lost in Britain through back pain) because they believe back pain is a 'skiver's charter' for casual absence or for the avoidance of certain tasks. On the other hand, some people with a highly developed sense of responsibility to work may be reluctant to take adequate time off. Many doctors would consider this attitude foolhardy. Some, however, would recommend a speedy return to work as part of the philosophy of confronting pain rather than giving in to it.

The problem of knowledge

One of the difficulties about curing back pain is that diagnosis is problematic: a great number of possible causes may manifest themselves as back pain. There is also the problem of why pain persists with no structural causes. There is a tendency to attribute most back pain to the minority of causes that are understood. This is compounded by the fact that most backaches get better spontaneously and therefore most cures 'work' so most experts can point to their successes as proof of the truth of their theories.

Improvements in the prevention and treatment of back trouble can only come after an increase in knowledge. We all know that machines must be oiled, maintained and used sensibly, to keep them working as long as possible. Yet replacements can be obtained for worn-out machine parts – but our bones have to last us as long as 80 years or more, and most of them are irreplaceable. As a first step to finding out how not to misuse them, it is worth getting to know how the back is constructed, and some of the ways in which it can be damaged.

CHAPTER 2

STRUCTURES OF THE BACK

THE spine has three main functions:

- it is the main support of the whole skeleton
- it protects the vital and vulnerable spinal cord
- it provides attachment points for muscles.

The bones of the spine

The spine is composed of 26 bones; 24 of these are separate vertebrae stacked on top of each other to form a column. They are graduated in size, so that the column is narrowest at the top, where the skull is balanced on it, and widest at the base, where it is balanced on the bony pelvis.

The spine is divided into five regions. Starting at the top, the first seven bones are cervical (neck) vertebrae. Next come the 12 thoracic (chest) vertebrae, each of them attached to a rib on each side, and the five lumbar vertebrae. Below them lies the sacrum, a curved wedge-shaped bone, which fits between the two hip bones of the pelvis; it consists of five sacral vertebrae fused together. A vestigial tail, the coccyx, composed of four tiny coccygeal vertebrae fused together, forms the thin end of the wedge.

A straight back?

The spinal column is not, as one might suppose, straight as a pillar: it has four curves. The cervical vertebrae curve forward, and so do the lumbar ones (producing the hollow of the back).

The spine

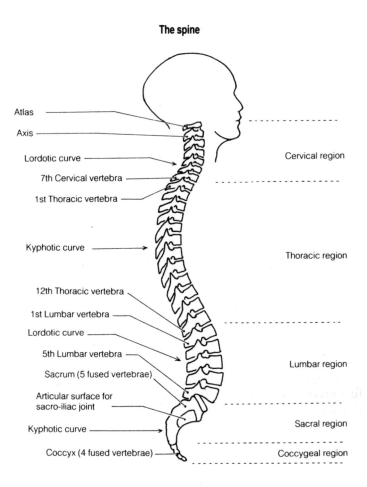

Atlas

Axis

Lordotic curve

7th Cervical vertebra

1st Thoracic vertebra

Cervical region

Kyphotic curve

Thoracic region

12th Thoracic vertebra

1st Lumbar vertebra

Lordotic curve

5th Lumbar vertebra

Sacrum (5 fused vertebrae)

Articular surface for
sacro-iliac joint

Kyphotic curve

Coccyx (4 fused vertebrae)

Lumbar region

Sacral region

Coccygeal region

The medical name for such a forward curve is lordosis. The thoracic vertebrae curve backwards, medically called a kyphosis, making a hollow for the chest; the sacrum with the coccyx also makes a backward curve. These natural curves make the spine more efficient at absorbing shocks and stresses.

The vertebrae

No two vertebrae are identical in shape or size, but all have a roughly similar outline. Except for the first two cervical vertebrae on which the head swivels and tilts, each vertebra has a solid block called the vertebral body, facing towards the front of the trunk. The rest of the vertebra is called the neural arch, and points towards the back. The arch is made up of several bony protrusions: two struts called pedicles jut out directly from the body. From these project a pair of sideways-pointing protrusions called the transverse processes. There are two more pairs of protrusions: the superior articular processes point upwards, the inferior articular processes point downwards.

These processes have oval, smooth cartilage-covered areas, called facets, which meet the corresponding surfaces above and below to form joints, called apophyseal joints or facet joints. Each vertebra is joined to the one above and the one below: each inferior articular process forms a joint with the superior process of the vertebra below it, and so on down the line. Like many other joints in the body, these vertebral joints are enclosed in capsules lined with a moist membrane called the synovium, which is lubricated with synovial fluid.

At the back of the neural arch is a protrusion called the spinous process. The bony layers between it and the rest of the arch, one on each side, are called laminae. The spinous processes are the knobs you can feel when you run your fingers down someone's spine.

The whole series of arches, stacked on top of each other, form a bony channel, down which passes the spinal cord, continuing from the base of the brain to the level of the first lumbar vertebra.

Intervertebral discs

The vertebral bodies are the weight-carrying parts of the vertebrae. They are separated by intervertebral discs, of which there

Lumbar vertebra

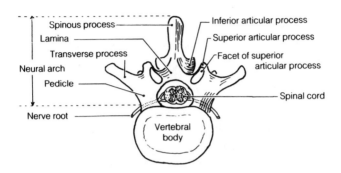

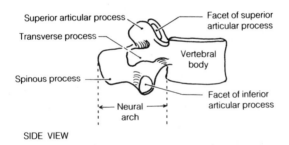

SIDE VIEW

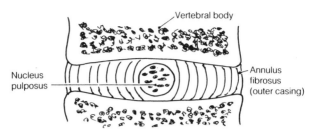

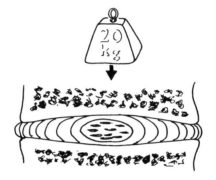

Disc when person is standing relaxed, with no loading

Disc when person is standing up carrying a heavy load

are 23 – one between every adjoining pair of vertebral bodies. In normal use, these discs are very efficient shock-absorbers; without them every step and movement would jar. The disc is a very tough structure. Inside a strong fibrous casing (annulus fibrosus) there is a pulpy gelatinous substance (nucleus pulposus), soft yet firm, and reinforced with strands of fibre. The disc has no blood and very little nerve supply, and consists mostly of water. During daily activity, the pressures on the spine force some fluid from the discs into the vertebral bodies. This is reabsorbed by the discs during relaxation, so that people actually become slightly shorter in the course of the day, and taller during the night. As people grow older, the discs lose some of their fluid content permanently and become thinner.

The spine and movement

Altogether there are 149 joints in the spine. As well as those which link the vertebrae to each other, there are those which link the spine to other structures. For instance, the first cervical vertebra is joined to the part of the skull called the occiput, and the sacrum is joined to the parts of the hip bones known as the ilia, forming the two sacroiliac joints. The ribs are joined to the transverse processes of the thoracic vertebrae.

The bony basin of the pelvis holds and protects many vital soft structures in the abdomen, such as the intestines and the female reproductive organs. Being articulated with the hip joints, it transfers weight down the legs to the feet. The tilt of the pelvis is an important factor for the balance of the spine.

The individual shapes of the vertebrae govern the direction of their movements, permitting certain movements and not others. For example, the first cervical vertebra (called the atlas), allows the head to nod backwards and forwards, and to tilt sideways. The second (called the axis) has a knob which fits into a socket through the atlas into the base of the skull: it allows the head to rotate, that is to turn to the left and right.

The thoracic vertebrae also allow backward, forward and sideways movement, and most of them also permit rotation – but only to a limited extent, because they are anchored to the rib cage. The lumbar vertebrae permit backward, forward and sideways movement only.

Ligaments

Wherever two bones form a joint, the two ends are bound together by fibrous bands or fibrous sheets. These are called ligaments, and are very strong, mostly inelastic but with some 'give'. The fibres of each ligament are aligned along the lines of force occurring at that joint, and control movement by allowing it only in a certain direction.

The ligaments of the vertebral column are of various types. The main ones are the longitudinal ligaments, long bands which run down the length of the spinal column, before and behind and to the sides of it. Other ones connect the processes of adjacent vertebrae, or connect the spine to other structures, such as the pelvis and the rib cage. The ligamentum flavum (yellow ligament) lines the back of the spinal canal, connecting the laminae of the arches; it is more elastic than other ligaments in the spine.

Three vertebrae of the lumbar spine

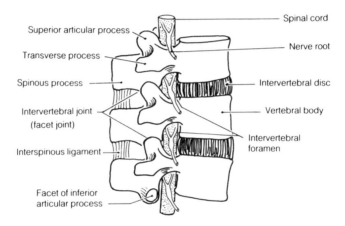

Superior articular process

Transverse process

Spinous process

Intervertebral joint
(facet joint)

Interspinous ligament

Facet of inferior
articular process

Spinal cord

Nerve root

Intervertebral disc

Vertebral body

Intervertebral
foramen

An intervertebral foramen is formed by the gap between the
pedicles of immediately adjacent vertebrae

The spinal canal

This is the conduit through which the spinal cord passes. It is formed by the backs of the vertebral bodies and the vertebral arches, and protects the spinal cord. The cord is surrounded by cerebro-spinal fluid, and encased in the dural tube which is made up of three tubular membranes, one inside the other. The dural tube descends all the way to the sacrum, though the spinal cord ends in the upper lumbar region.

The spinal cord is an extension of the brain, and is the trunk road of the nervous system, conveying information from the brain to all regions of the body and back again, by means of nerve roots which branch out from it.

At the level of each vertebra, the nerve roots emerge through chinks, known as intervertebral foramina, between adjacent pedicles, one on each side of each vertebra. Each nerve root is enclosed in a dural sleeve. From all these pairs of nerve roots a vast network of nerves branches out throughout the whole body.

Since the spinal cord stops short at the first lumbar vertebra, there is a sheaf of pairs of nerve roots passing downwards from the lower segments of the spinal cord to reach their respective foramina. This sheaf is called the cauda equina, the horse's tail, because that is what it looks like.

The network of nerves which originate in the nerve roots has a pattern of distribution which is much the same for everyone, with only minor individual deviations. It is therefore possible to trace a pain sensation in any part of the body, caused by a compressed nerve root, back to its point of origin in the spine. For example, a pain in the big toe that is caused by a compressed nerve must originate in the last two lumbar vertebrae or the upper part of the sacrum – nowhere else in the spine.

The spinal cord is not easily injured, except through fracture or dislocation of the spine or when the cord is penetrated by sharp instruments, bullets or shrapnel. In normal circumstances, the spinal canal and its contents are protected from injury by bone and ligaments and muscle.

The spinal canal changes its length with spinal movement. When you bend sideways, it becomes longer on one side than the other. On bending forwards and flexing the spine, the whole canal lengthens, more so behind than in front. The change in length in the cervical and lumber regions may be as much as 25 per cent, and the contents of the spinal canal adapt accordingly. When the spine is bent back and arched, the intervertebral discs tend to bulge forwards and the ligaments at the back of the spinal canal slacken.

In the course of vertebral movements, the gaps between each pair of vertebrae (the intervertebral foramina) open and close, as the neighbouring vertebral arches move closer together or separate, and the nerve roots move inside the foramina.

Muscles

Muscles are the fleshy part of the body and consist of long, thin fibres, bound together in bundles by connective tissue, and supplied with blood and nerves. What is remarkable about these fibres is that they can become shorter in response to a stimulus. The shortening is caused by protein filaments inside the cells which pull against each other; on relaxation, the muscles are pulled back into their original position, by gravity or by the action of other muscles. Sometimes the cells are unable to relax their hold – this involuntary contraction of a muscle is called a spasm and may be caused by pain.

There are, roughly speaking, two types of muscle: the involuntary and the voluntary. The heart and the hollow organs (digestive system, uterus, blood vessels, etc.) are of the first sort. They work without conscious control while life lasts – you do not need to instruct your heart to beat. The voluntary muscles are mostly under conscious control, so that it is for you to decide to move your limbs, for example; but you do not, of course, have to plan the movements of each muscle. When you decide to bend your knees, for instance, reflex actions determine the different movements of the several different muscles which this entails, and you neither know, nor need to know which ones they are.

The voluntary muscles also respond to various stimuli through reflex actions – when you touch a hot stove, messages racing along the nerves will jerk away your hand faster than thought.

Because they can be controlled, the voluntary muscles can be trained to work more efficiently. With suitable training, the nervous system learns how to recruit muscle fibres more rapidly and more precisely, and the muscles themselves become stronger and bigger and more capable of clearing away the waste products of their activity, so that they can continue working for longer. If they are not exercised, they waste away quickly.

The action of a muscle is to develop tension between two points on the skeleton, so as to draw them together or prevent their being pulled apart or control the rate at which they are being pulled apart. Without muscular control, the spine is much less stable – as in an unconscious person.

The muscles which control the spine are those of the back and neck and the abdominal muscles.

The muscles of the back

There are several layers of back muscles, their shape being different in each layer. No muscle crosses the mid-line demarcated by the vertebral column – for every muscle on one side of the back there is a matching one on the other side. Their points of attachment to the spine are the transverse and spinous processes of the vertebrae.

The largest back muscles are those in the topmost layer. They are triangular, extending in diagonal sheets across either side of the back, and they attach the spinous processes of the backbone to the shoulder blade and shoulder joints. These muscles hold the whole body steady when you are using your arms and legs to lift heavy weights.

The deeper layers are long, strap-shaped muscles extending vertically along the vertebral column. Most of them originate at a small area on the back of the pelvis, fanning out to attach themselves to various ribs as well as to vertebrae, and up to the head. This 'railway junction' on the pelvis is a common site of low back pain, which in some cases is the result of inflammation of these muscle origins.

At the deepest layers, the muscles are short and thick, extending only from one vertebra to the next, or its two or three neighbours, and keeping these bones aligned with each other; but they will only stay aligned if the muscles on either side are equally strong. If these small muscles go into spasm on one side only at a particular level, the total posture is affected.

The abdominal muscles

These share the task of keeping the spine upright by exerting a pull down the front of the trunk that counterbalances that exerted by the back muscles. They also help the spine to bend, by pulling the front of the rib cage closer to the pelvis.

Abdominal muscles also control twisting actions between the shoulders and the pelvis – no golfer could do without them – and they are used when pushing, and for holding the posture when leaning backwards. When the body is bent sideways, they share the work with the back muscles on that side.

A muscle called psoas (from the greek for loin) passes from the lumbar vertebral bodies, round the pelvis, and over each hip-joint to the upper end of each thigh–bone. It contracts when you sit up from lying down. When it is active, it pulls on the lumbar vertebrae, compressing the discs.

There is also an indirect mechanism by which the abdominal muscles support the spine. When a weight is being lifted, these muscles, in conjunction with the back muscles and the other muscles forming the abdominal cavity, tighten automatically. This increases the pressure inside the cavity, making it loadbearing (in the same way that inflating a balloon makes it able to support a weight), and as the compressed abdomen presses against the spine, it absorbs some of the load on the spine, and helps the back to straighten up.

Weight-lifters deliberately increase their intra-abdominal pressure by wearing a special belt. For ordinary people, it is enough to keep the abdominal muscles in good condition: this is very important for preventing backache.

What happens when you bend

When you start to lean forwards, the muscles of the back become active and tensed in order to counter the effects of gravity on the upper half of the body which is now forward of the hips, so that the trunk is cantilevered from the pelvis. There is a compensatory movement of the hips backwards to maintain the line of gravity within the base of support. On further bending, however, as the hands pass the level of the knees, the back muscles stop working and the strain is taken by the ligaments. The restraint on the spine by either muscles or ligaments imposes a force on it which

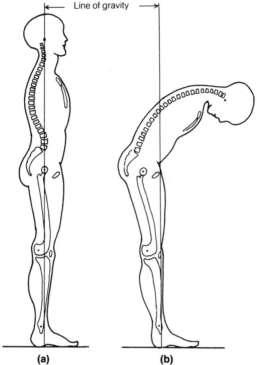

(a) Line of gravity through the erect body. The disc spaces are approximately even in width from front to back

(b) When you bend forward the discs are narrower at the front than at the back, and the length of the spinal canal between the cervical and lumbar regions can increase by up to 25%

(Note that in flexing the torso we move our legs backwards so that the pelvis is behind the line of gravity through the erect body; otherwise the weight of the torso would cause us to fall forwards.)

compresses the vertebral bodies and discs. The muscles of the hip, thigh and back are strongly active when holding the trunk in the forward position, and have to become even more active to bring the body upright again. The muscles do not resume their work until the hips are again at right angles.

Tendons and fascia

The muscles in the arms and legs are attached to the bones by means of tendons (sinews) which are tough, fibrous elongations of the muscle fibres. The muscles attached to the vertebrae are not always connected by tendons; in some places very tough, thin sheets of connective tissue, called fascia, connect the muscles to the vertebrae. A big band of fascia runs down the neck, becoming rectangular across the nape. There is another big, rectangular sheet of fascia at waist level. When the muscles are working strongly, the fascia and tendons take the strain at the point where they are attached to the bone.

CHAPTER 3

How the damage is done

THE various structures of the human back together form a complex piece of engineering. The backbone at one end is balanced on a tilting pelvis, and the other holds up a heavy head; at the same time it provides support for the movement of the arms and legs.

The skeletal system forms a mechanism which, although not properly ossified, is functionally complete at birth; it goes into full operation whenever a baby learns to stand and walk upright. The bones consolidate their shape during the teenage years and, under ideal conditions, should work perfectly for a lifetime. In practice, as we know, it is often otherwise. There are a great many ways in which the balance of the mechanism can be disturbed. Sometimes the damage is done all in an instant, as the result of a single violent incident. At other times, it is cumulative, the conclusion of a long series of small stresses. It has been thought that parts of the back, like those of any domestic appliance, may simply wear out through constant use. But there is no very good evidence for this: the resilience of most of the human body tends to belie such notions.

Stress on the spine

The spine can never be at rest while life lasts, because the thoracic vertebrae, which are attached to the rib cage, move with every breath, straightening as you breathe in and flexing forward as you breathe out.

The spine plays a part in the movements of most other parts of the body. Moving the head in relation to the chest causes movement in the cervical and upper thoracic vertebrae; moving the arms also moves the thoracic spine; the lumbar spine is involved in movements of the upper part of the trunk in relation to the pelvis, and in moving the legs.

The spine and gravity

The vertical force exerted on the human body by gravity varies according to the position the body assumes. Gravity is least stressful in the lying-down position, and the stress is well distributed in moving on all fours (which is one reason why back pain victims sometimes have to revert to crawling); but the erect stance of *homo sapiens* is maintained in defiance of gravity, and the gravitational load exerted on the head, arms and upper trunk is taken mainly by the vertebral bodies, and the intervertebral discs. (Back problems are, however, not exclusive to those who happen to stand erect. There is a popular misconception that if only we walked on all fours, we would have no back problems. But some animals undoubtedly do have back troubles: horses, dogs – especially dachshunds.)

The muscles, too, undergo gravitational stress, depending on the direction of movement. In bending, the downward movement of the trunk is helped by gravity, with the muscles and ligaments controlling and limiting the descent; in straightening up, the muscles must do all the work, against gravity, but once the upright position is achieved, they do not need to work very hard to maintain it.

The effects of movement

Any muscular activity and movement causes some increase in spinal stress. If you stand on the bathroom scales and watch the pointer while you raise your arms, you will see it move up. The force needed to lift the arms is passed down your spine to your feet and (via the scales) to the floor. The same is true of every other activity – pushing, pulling, carrying, getting up, sitting down.

Body movements that are caused by outside forces also cause stress on the spine. Most forms of transport, from horses and bicycles to trains and buses, bounce and jolt the human frame; apart from jolts and jars, most people occasionally stumble or fall. The force of all such vibrations is imparted to and resisted by the spine, but in most cases it suffers no serious injury, because of its capacity for absorbing shocks. It converts the energy into movement by going with the impact instead of resisting it and alters the quality of the applied force, so that it is less likely to cause injury.

The function of converting force into movement is a vital one. Unless some of the applied energy can be quickly converted into movement, it will break bones or cause other injury. In young and supple people, much more movement can be produced than in someone old and stiff, and they can therefore take more punishment than the elderly. As well as being more mobile, the structures in a young spine can bend or change shape more readily in response to loads and muscular tension. This is why the young are better than old people at 'taking' forces and reducing them.

Spinal functions also include a safety mechanism: namely, protective backache or pain. Pain is information and mainly of value in giving warning of postural stress. It is not so effective at preventing injury caused when something proves too heavy to lift or will not move because it is, unexpectedly, stuck – then the pain may come too late.

Damage to the discs

Intervertebral discs are not easily injured. The gel-like nucleus of the disc allows it to change shape, rather like a cushion that is sat on, in response to pressures that are exerted on it. The tightly-woven fibres of the outer casing, the annulus, are very strong and moderately elastic, so that, like a cushion cover, it is able to accommodate, without tearing, most changes in the shape of its contents. However, although strong, it is not invulnerable. It may tear if subjected to a twisting action, that is, any movement in which the vertebrae above and below the disc are made to rotate in opposite directions. This sort of injury can be caused by an untoward movement in the course of vigorous exercise, for instance, or through lifting a heavy object awkwardly. It is most

Damage to an intervertebral disc

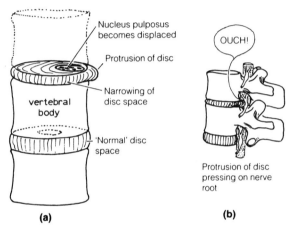

(a) When an intervertebral disc is damaged by injury, disease or faulty posture the fibres of annulus fibrosus become weakened and allow the disc to protrude at the edge

(b) If the protrusion encroaches upon the spinal canal or an intervertebral foramen it could press upon a nerve root and cause severe pain likely to happen when the trunk is bent forward: in this position the lumbar facet joints are less effective at preventing rotation.

When the tear is very severe, the pulpy nucleus of the disc is forced out by the pressure of the vertebrae above the tear (like toothpaste squeezed out of a tube), and protrudes out of the tear. Such an injury is rare. If the outer casing does not tear, the nucleus will remain contained within the casing, but its pressure may cause the disc to bulge outwards.

Prolapsed disc

If the protrusion or the bulge does not press on any sensitive structures there are no symptoms, because the disc has almost no nerve supply of its own. If the bulge presses against one of the ligaments which bind the spine together, or against a nerve root, the pain can be intense. This condition, called a prolapsed disc, is what is popularly, but incorrectly, called a slipped disc. A disc cannot, in fact, slip out of place, because its fibres are knitted into the bone of the adjacent vertebral bodies.

Any disc may suffer a prolapse but, for reasons that are not well understood, those most frequently affected are the last two in the lumbar spine – the one that lies between the fourth and fifth lumbar vertebrae and the one between the fifth and the sacrum. One reason why discs at those sites become affected may be because those are the points of maximum movement for the lumbar spine.

The commonest direction for a prolapse is backwards and sideways. The symptoms arise from the irritation of the sensitive structures and the associated inflammation, similar to the inflammation following any injury. This develops over a day or so, and spreads to involve other tissues at the same vertebral level. It may cause back pain or sciatic pain (down the leg), depending on whether it affects the tissues of the spine or of the nerve root, or both.

Prolapsed discs resulting from violent injury are probably likeliest to occur in young people who are most apt to go in for strenuous games, 'working out', disco dancing, and so forth; young nurses also have a fairly high rate of disc injury, through lifting and turning patients.

In middle-aged people, however, it is gradual degeneration of the casing of the disc, rather than violent exercise, that is the commonest cause of disc prolapse. The fibrous outer casing of the disc gradually weakens and grows stiffer, developing cracks through which the nucleus can leak out.

As a small compensation, disc prolapse becomes much less common once middle age is past and this, too, is due to degenerative changes. The nucleus, losing much of its moisture, shrinks considerably, and though it may spread out, it is less apt to leak out of the casing. However, this change brings its own problems, as the disc loses some of its shock-absorbing ability.

Damage to the bones

The vertebrae, like any other bones, can be fractured by a blow, accidental or deliberate – a car crash, a fall from a height, a bullet may chip one of the vertebrae, or even detach a fragment. Too vigorous exercise may do the same: if a tendon attached to one of the transverse processes is overstretched, it may come away, taking a piece of the bone with it. Violent, unskilled physical effort may also cause microscopic fractures in the cartilage covering the flat sides of the vertebral bodies.

Compression forces which are too powerful for the discs to absorb – for instance, the violent jolt of a leap from a height, as in a poor parachute landing – may cause a crush fracture of a vertebra: shattering the vertebral body or forcing it out of shape, or breaking off the transverse processes.

Spinal fractures are often, but not invariably, painful; they usually mend with rest. A crush fracture may displace part of a vertebra so as to produce a slight hump that can be seen and felt. Sometimes an X-ray discloses bone damage of which the owner of the spine was unaware, and which gave no trouble. However, the most serious fractures, those that damage the spinal cord, can cause paralysis below the site of the injury.

Spondylolysis

A fracture or crack of the vertebral arch in the lower lumbar spine is called spondylolysis. It may happen either suddenly or gradually as the culmination of a series of repeated strains – rather like a fatigue fracture in metal; or as a result of a congenital defect. It often causes no symptoms and a person may have it all his life without knowing.

Spondylolisthesis

This is a condition in which a vertebra slips forward out of alignment with the part of the spine below it. It commonly arises in the fourth or the fifth lumbar vertebra, so that all the rest of the spine moves forward out of line with the sacrum. The usual cause is a defect or crack of the neural arch (spondylolysis), which causes the facet joints of the articular processes, which normally hold the vertebrae in line, to loosen their hold.

Much less commonly, the slippage may be in a backwards direction; it is then called retrolisthesis.

The causes of the trouble may come from a hereditary weakness of the neural arch: it seems to run in some families and some races, being common among Eskimos. It may, however arise from injury, such as a heavy fall on to one's behind; or from constant stress, as in the case of athletes and gymnasts; or simply from wear and tear in middle age.

In spondylolisthesis the damage, unlike many vertebral fractures, does not heal spontaneously, perhaps because the lumbar spine has a natural forward curve.

There may be severe pain, if deformation of the neural arch or the displacement of a vertebral body causes pressure on a nerve; or if the slippage damages the disc fibres and brings about a prolapse.

Cumulative damage

However, most damage to the bones of the spine is cumulative. The spine is a symmetrical structure, and can be damaged by stress that is unequally distributed. When the vertebral bodies are continually made to bear uneven stresses by being loaded more heavily on one side than on the other, wear and tear causes irregular shaping of the bone material.

Scoliosis

This is the name of a sideways curvature of the vertebral column. It may be a congenital condition, or the result of muscular weakness on one side of the spine, or the consequence of bone disease in childhood. Misalignment of the shoulders and hips, with one appearing higher than the other, is a common sign of scoliosis; women who have this problem cannot get their hemlines to hang straight.

If this condition is detected in childhood, when the bones are growing, it should not be ignored: treatment by splinting or bracing may be required to prevent the child from growing up badly deformed. If mild, the condition may resolve without treatment. Spinal surgery may be advised in severe cases.

A less conspicuous type of scoliosis occurs in people who are born with one leg slightly shorter than the other. Quite often they do not walk with a limp, having become used to compensating for the inequality by curving the spine slightly towards the longer leg: in this way they keep the trunk level.

When the vertebral column bends sideways, the vertebrae automatically rotate slightly to accommodate the posture; this is unlikely to cause any trouble in the short term. However, a scoliotic spine is more liable to injury than a normal one, because the curvature makes it harder for the vertebrae to rearrange themselves as demanded by all the activities of daily life. They may therefore lock or jam in one position. In the long term, they wear down more on one side than on the other, because the stresses on them are unequal, with resulting strain on the neighbouring joints and muscles, perhaps causing pain.

Another type of scoliosis is temporary, and occurs in people suffering from a prolapsed disc, or some other painful back problem. Their normal posture being painful, they instinctively adjust the position of the vertebrae to achieve a more comfortable position. This may bring its own problems, because the spine is then unbalanced, but the scoliosis should disappear when the pain does.

Damage to the joints and ligaments

The spine is organised so precisely that it is hardly possible to damage any one of its components without affecting all the rest, even though the effect of this may not become apparent for a long time.

Anything that alters the shape or position of the vertebrae causes additional stress on the facet joints which help to keep the vertebrae in place, and they, in turn, then exert more stress on the muscles and ligaments.

When all the joints of the spine are fully mobile, the sum of all the little movements that they are able to perform amounts to a wide range of activity – all that anyone should ever need. But if some of these joints should become stiff – something that one might be unaware of at the time – the other joints find it more difficult to carry out their normal range of movements. This, in turn, places the adjoining muscles at a disadvantage, causing them to go into spasm, which then puts stress on the work of the other muscle groups in the region.

Moreover, many people go in for daily activities which require the spine to move in ways which are anatomically unwise. Many so-called keep-fit exercises also demand movements which the spine is not constructed to perform, and which are stressful to the joints.

A serious injury is 'whiplash' (which may be caused in a car accident) when, as the result of impact, the head is violently jerked forwards or backwards and the neck ligaments severely strained or even torn.

At the lower end of the spine, the pelvis is joined to the sacrum by the sacroiliac joints, reinforced by strong ligaments, which may, however, be damaged by a sudden jolt: by sitting down very hard, or by violent exercise that involves a twisting motion. A commoner reason for trouble there is reserved for mothers. Towards the end of pregnancy, hormonal action softens these ligaments, in order to allow easier passage to the baby's head through the pelvic ring, and this makes the sacroiliac joints prone to injury. Once the baby is born, the ligaments tighten again over a period of several months.

However, if there is additional strain when the joint is loosened, or if there are frequent pregnancies, the ligaments joining the two bones may never quite recover their original immobility.

Misaligned joints

The facet joints which unite each vertebra to its immediate neighbours may be jerked out of alignment by severe sudden stress, such as a twisting movement: this is called subluxation. A still more violent movement may pull the bones even farther apart so that the joint becomes unstable; this is called dislocation. It is uncommon unless there is severe force. Subluxation may also be the result of growing older. The intervertebral discs flatten out as they lose their moisture, so that the spine becomes shorter, and the ligaments which support it become slack. This may allow some play in the facet joints, with a greater chance of misalignment.

Both types of injury, subluxation and dislocation, are more likely to occur when the body is bent over and the joints are already undergoing tension.

In either case, there is some tearing of the ligaments which bind the facets together, and which are part of the synovial capsule enclosing the joint. There may be some internal bleeding; the irritated capsule becomes inflamed and swollen, and there is pain.

Stress on the ligaments

The ligaments in an adult have very little elasticity. They can be strained, that is, over-stretched by violent action, usually at their points of attachment to the bone. They can also tear, usually in the direction in which their fibres are weakest. Torn ligaments heal rather slowly (more slowly than bone).

Ligaments do not have blood vessels within; any bleeding which occurs when a ligament is torn comes from the surrounding tissues. This results in the formation of fibrin, protein fibres which form new tissue to mend the damage. Often this causes scar tissue to form along the line of the mend (rather like excess glue along the cracks in repaired china), and this may adhere to the surrounding tissues, hampering the movement of the ligament. Further strain may wrench and tear these adhesions, causing more inflammation, and pain.

Joints at risk

The little facet joints at the side of the spine take more mechanical strain from unequal stresses on the spine than the main intervertebral joint itself. The subsequent inflammation is a common cause of low back pain, particularly the type that gets worse with exercise or as the day goes on.

The facet joints in the lower lumbar spine have the function of preventing the vertebrae from rotating, and so are especially vulnerable to damage from twisting movements, but joint injuries may occur anywhere along the spine.

At the upper end, strain on the cervical vertebrae can send the neck muscles into spasm, producing a 'stiff neck' (called torticollis, or wry-neck). This usually gets better in a short time when the spasm decontracts.

Damage to the muscles and tendons

The muscles which support the spine and control its movements are liable to injury by the same stresses that damage the vertebrae and joints. Muscular injury may be related to postural stress, or to excessive or miscalculated effort.

An example is bending with a sudden jerking movement without allowing the back muscles to arrange themselves for coordinated effort. This can cause excessive strain to the muscles which have the job of controlling bending movements of the spine.

Any unaccustomed effort can injure a muscle; keep-fit and other exercises which do not begin with a warm-up period can result in aching muscles or even injury. People who rashly dig the whole garden after a winter's inactivity are likely to suffer for it.

Another way to do damage is to lift heavy or awkwardly placed loads, particularly if this involves bending or off-centre one-armed efforts, or sideways twisting.

Muscular spasm: the pain/spasm cycle

In most parts of the body, following injury or pain, the involuntary response of the surrounding muscles is to contract in a spasm, clasping the hurting part as in a vice. This prevents it from being used any further, and so protects it, but it also impedes the blood circulation. If the pain was caused by pressure on a nerve, the spasm reinforces the pressure, setting up a kind of vicious cycle. For the damage to be repaired, and the function in the damaged part to be restored, the muscular spasm must first relax.

Muscles at risk

Each movement of a joint is a harmony of different muscle actions. Some muscles shorten to produce the movement. Other opposing muscles allow themselves to be lengthened to control the movement, a third set of muscles is busy cancelling out unwanted associated movements to enhance the performance, and a fourth set of muscles is holding the body fixed and firm to provide a solid foundation on which movements can take place. If the muscles around some of the vertebrae were to jerk and tug in opposite directions, there would be pain and muscle spasm, causing these vertebrae to be pulled and twisted even more. Ligaments and tendons could be damaged, and the muscle tissue become inflamed. One example of such unbalanced action is twisting oneself out of a car seat while carrying a heavy bag, or manoeuvring an infant into a car seat in the rear of a two-door car.

It is important for the muscles to be trained and worked equally on both sides of the vertebral column. If an action uses mostly the muscles on one side, a deliberate effort should be made to follow that action with another that uses the muscles on the other side. For instance, when polishing, a spell of using the right arm should be followed by an equally long spell of using the left arm – or vice versa.

Asymmetrical stressing is particularly damaging in childhood, when the bones are growing; while symmetrical pressure encourages the bone to become dense and strong. Any weights that are carried should be evenly balanced on both sides of the body, with a straight back.

Injured muscles can be extremely painful, but as a rule they recover completely with no treatment other than rest. Healing may be total but where it is accompanied by shortening of the muscles, rendering the structures more vulnerable, some therapy – gradual stretching – will help.

Muscle pain from postural stress

Most people at one time or another experience the discomfort of aching muscles caused by adopting an awkward posture. For instance, holding a book at arm's length is hard work on the shoulder muscles, not because the book is heavy, but because it is exerting a leverage at the end of the long arm, and this greatly magnifies its weight. In contrast, when that leverage is removed by simply letting the arm hang, the task is easy. Leaning forwards over a bench imposes the same kind of stress on the muscles of the back, for then the weight of the head and trunk is exerting leverage through the spine on the hips and lower back of up to four or five times as much as when the body is upright. If these postures are sustained, discomfort and pain may result. As a general principle, the more intense the muscle tension, the sooner the discomfort begins. It is therefore important to change postures frequently, to share the load of any task between all the muscles that may reasonably be harnessed to help, and to take adequate rest breaks. A series of short routine actions can also cause muscle tension and postural fatigue if repeated too often, as in assembly-line work in a factory.

The bad design of some equipment and furniture used in work, both domestic and outside the house, readily causes muscular stress in the user. It is also true that many people let themselves in for unnecessary muscular ache, in the back and neck muscles and elsewhere, by adopting a bad posture: such as sitting slumped in a chair, or humped over a desk.

Pain in the back muscles caused by postural stress can generally be relieved by rest and/or change of position and postural retraining. In extreme cases, it may become chronic and require treatment. Also, when a neighbouring part of the spine is painful and inflamed, the back muscles may be held taut to guard against a painful movement, and this in turn may fatigue them and make them ache. The additional pain resulting from this tightening of the muscles can be a considerable component of the pain experienced. Consciously trying to relax can help; if not, treatment of the inflamed condition will be needed to relieve the soreness in the muscles.

Not all muscular pain is caused by postural stress. Anxiety and frustration can give rise to muscular tension. If the frustration has no outlet or the anxiety is not relieved, muscular pain can occur. Tension in the shoulders and neck can also produce headaches.

CHAPTER 4

AGEING AND DEGENERATIVE CHANGE

As one gets older, the whole spine tends to become stiffer. Not only is the total range of movement reduced, but the tissues in the spine are stiffer and change shape less readily, which reduces their shock-absorbing capacity.

To some extent, degenerative change can produce similar effects locally in individual joints. A completely degenerated intervertebral joint – disc, ligaments and joint facets – is stiff, fibrous, and narrow.

Degenerative change can start in one's teens, but the likelihood of it increases with age. It differs from the ageing process, however, in that ageing affects the spine as a whole, while degeneration generally begins in a single intervertebral segment. There may be advanced degenerative change in just one site, with apparently normal discs and joints above and below it.

Degeneration may begin in the disc itself, or in the joints or ligaments – particularly the interspinous ligaments which join the vertebrae.

Degenerative change tends to begin much earlier in people who do heavy unskilled manual labour. It can also start early in people who go in for strenuous forms of exercise – but some experienced weightlifters show no more degenerative change than sedentary workers. It seems that violent exertions and unskilled efforts are most likely to cause minor damage to the cartilage between discs and vertebral bodies, or to the ligaments. If they are repeated often, there is a cumulative effect leading to degeneration, even though at the time each injury felt no worse than a momentary jarring. There is also some evidence that prolonged awkward posture may lead to such damage.

Back pain and degeneration do not invariably go together; they do not necessarily bear any relationship to each other. Plenty of people undergo major degenerative changes in their spine without ever suffering from back pain.

Disc degeneration

A completely degenerated disc is much thinner than a normal one. On an X-ray, this shows up as a narrowing of the space between vertebral bodies, since the disc itself does not show on X-rays. As well as being flattened, it is stiff and fibrous. At this stage it is unlikely to cause back pain. When the degenerative process has reached this stage of stiffness, and the nucleus has dried out, there is much less risk of prolapse, and the system is stable.

It is in the earlier stages of degeneration that disc injuries and pain are more likely. The disc is much weaker than it was formerly, and much readier to bulge. It can therefore become the source of repeated back trouble. Mechanically, it can no longer restrain the shearing forces between the vertebral bodies as efficiently as it once did, and therefore the joints and ligaments may have to resist greater strains than they are designed for.

A sign of degenerative change is the appearance of small ruptures in the annulus fibrosus (the outer casing) and the pulpy nucleus tends to spread through these. It is at this stage that some people undergo a disc prolapse which can cause trouble.

Ligament degeneration

Ligaments also undergo degenerative changes. The interspinous ligaments often begin to degenerate in people whose spine has become so stiff that they can no longer bend forwards. The ligaments become somewhat narrower, and their structure can become disorganised by ruptures and cavities. They then become a likely source of pain and local tenderness. These changes can occur at one ligament or a series of ligaments involving various levels of the spine.

Degeneration also affects the ligamentum flavum (the more elastic ligament which lines the back of the spinal canal), particularly when the spine has become stiff, and the ligament is no longer stretched normally. It becomes more fibrous, loses its elasticity, and can become a source of pain.

Joint degeneration

When the spinal joints are subjected to abnormal wear and tear, such as repeated sprains, the cartilage which lines the joint facets becomes thinner and more fibrous, and the articular processes tend to become thicker where they are attached to the capsule of the joint. This thickening reduces the space in the spinal canal and the intervertebral gaps. Degenerated facet joints can become the site of back pain, and of pain felt over the buttock and down the thigh.

Osteophytosis

This is not a degenerative condition in its own right but may be a secondary manifestation to a degenerative disease. Osteophytosis is part of the healing of a fracture. It is the formation of osteophytes, bony growths or spurs, on bone, or fibrous tissue attached to bone. They are deposits of calcium, the material of bone; in the spine they form all round the edges of the flat sides of the vertebral bodies, and on the facet joints.

Osteophytosis is in fact a feature of osteoarthrosis (also called osteoarthritis), a degenerative disease of the joints, causing a thickening of the bone. (It should not be confused with rheumatoid arthritis, which is a very different and more distressing complaint.)

Although on X-ray osteophytes can look formidably hook-like, they usually cause trouble only if they happen to grow out into the chinks through which the nerve roots pass, or into the spinal canal itself: if nerve tissue is compressed, this can be very painful. Such problems are most likely to arise in the lumbar region, where the cauda equina, with its bundle of nerves, emerges from the dural tube.

Osteophytes can cause back trouble in people who have by nature a very narrow spinal canal. Where the spinal canal is trefoil shaped (rather than roughly round) the growth of osteophytes further reduces the space through which the nerve roots pass, and the person is likely to suffer from back problems.

CHAPTER 5

OTHER BACK PROBLEMS

THE kinds of back trouble that have been described so far derive from some dysfunction of the spine or from a congenital deformity, or from a violent injury, or from gradual deterioration with use and age.

There are other kinds of back trouble. Some of them affect the spine mainly or solely; others affect various parts of the body, the spine being just one of them. A third category includes disease which produces back pain without necessarily involving the spine.

Ankylosing spondylitis

This is a chronic inflammatory condition or arthritis, predominantly affecting spinal joints. It tends to run in families (but not always so that every member is afflicted). It affects men more than women, and symptoms often start young, in the teens. It is a systemic disease; the person feels ill when the disease is active, and other parts of the body (for example the eyes) may be affected.

In ankylosing spondylitis, the same process of laying down calcium deposits which creates osteophytes may continue to the point of fusing together some vertebrae, so that the spine in that region becomes completely stiff.

It starts usually in the lining of the sacroiliac joints and spreads gradually upwards to the other joints of the spine; it sometimes also spreads downwards into the hip joints and, more rarely, other leg joints. Over a period of time the inflammation may cause the ligaments of the joints to calcify, so that the joints become *ankylosed* (rigid) producing, in the worst cases, a spine locked permanently in a bowed posture. The ligaments joining the ribs to the spine may also harden, flattening the rib cage and making breathing difficult. This is one of the early symptoms. Others are pain and stiffness in the hip joints, which feel worst in the morning, because they are made worse by lying still and are relieved by movement. Painkillers and anti-inflammatory drugs as prescribed by the doctor will help considerably. Exercise is invaluable: it should be taught by a physiotherapist. Done regularly, it may help to keep the joints flexible and avoid severe deformity. Many patients take up squash, tennis, swimming and other sports and prefer this to the repetitive use of formal exercises over many years.

Arachnoiditis

This is an inflammation of the arachnoid mater, one of the three membranes making up the dural tube which sheathes the spinal cord, and the dural sleeves which sheathe the nerve roots. The inflammation causes the membrane to grow thicker and proliferate, particularly round the nerve roots, where they enter the dural sleeves. This crowds the nerves inside, so that they cannot move freely in and out of the sleeve. The result is back pain, and also pain down the arms and/or legs, with tingling or pins and needles.

Arachnoiditis can be caused by some infection involving the cerebro-spinal system, such as meningitis, and can also occur as the aftermath of surgery on the spine, through the formation of scar tissue inside the dural sleeves. Formerly, oil-based contrast dyes were used in X-raying the spine, and would sometimes cause arachnoiditis, but these are no longer used. There may be other causes, not yet identified. Recent investigations are suggesting that the sufferers tend to produce too much fibrin (protein formed in blood-clotting) and thus excessive scarring. There is at present no effective treatment, other than prescribing painkillers. It may prove that hormone treatment will be helpful in some circumstances.

Osteoporosis

This is a bone condition associated with growing old, and may affect any bone, not just those of the back. It takes the form of loss of bone material (calcium and minerals), making the bones fracture more easily. The spine tends to shrink in overall length, so that the person becomes shorter. In advanced cases, the affected vertebrae may collapse in a series of crush fractures, so that the sufferer develops a curvature of the spine, becoming round-shouldered. The 'dowager's hump' seen in elderly women may be caused in this way.

There is some association with the sex hormones, because osteoporosis is common in post-menopausal women and women whose ovaries have been removed. In them, it responds dramatically to treatment with oestrogen – hormone replacement therapy.

Physically active people are less likely to develop osteoporosis. Exercise is thought to have some protective function. Bone loss can be the result of prolonged immobility, and is one reason why doctors discourage patients from staying in bed longer than absolutely necessary. Astronauts spending weeks and months in space beyond the reach of earth's gravitational pull also suffer bone loss – but this is not yet a common hazard.

The loss of bone is not in itself painful, but there may be pain anywhere in the spine and in the joints between the spine and the ribs, as the spine adapts to its new conformation. Loss of spinal bone leading to crush fractures may lead to trapping of pain-sensitive structures, such as nerve roots.

A related but much less common complaint is osteomalacia, a softening of the bones caused by vitamin D deficiency in adults (in children the result is rickets). It is thought that osteoporosis and osteomalacia may respond to increased calcium and vitamin D in the diet. But this is in no way proven, and people should certainly not dose themselves with calcium supplements – these may even make you ill.

Paget's disease (osteitis deformans)

This is a bone disease of unknown origin, and may occur in any bone. It usually starts in middle age and is rarely found before the age of 60. The bones thicken and become denser, but also softer, tending to deform. If the disease is mild, as is often the case, and causes no symptoms, no treatment is given. In the spine, Paget's disease may cause pain through pressure on the nerve roots; painkillers may suffice.

Treatment, notably with calcitonin, a hormone which inhibits the excessive laying down of bone material, is very expensive and considered justifiable in only very few cases.

Rheumatoid arthritis

Although this disease predominantly affects the joints of the limbs, the spine may also be affected. It is a crippling disease of the synovial joints in any part of the body, affecting the synovium, the membrane which lines the joints. Its cause is not completely understood, but it is now believed that it may involve an auto-immune reaction – the body, turning against itself, producing antibodies against some of its own tissues. But the evidence that it is an auto-immune disease is controversial.

Attacks of rheumatoid arthritis take the form of inflammation of the joints, giving rise to aching and stiffness, especially in the mornings; in rare cases, it may be accompanied by fever. Attacks tend to recur and may finally leave the joints swollen and rigid.

Rheumatoid arthritis tends to start in the smaller joints, such as those of the fingers, and gradually spreads to the larger ones. In the spine, it tends first to affect the neck (sometimes the earliest symptom is neck pain) or the lumbar area. By the time the lumbar area is affected, the disease is considerably advanced, and the sufferer is probably already receiving treatment. So your first attack of back pain is highly unlikely to be rheumatoid arthritis: if it were, you would have had plenty of warning.

If you know that you have rheumatoid arthritis, avoid manipulative therapies such as those given by osteopaths and chiropractors. The ligaments between the first and second cervical vertebrae are often affected and sudden jerks of your head can provoke serious damage to the spinal cord.

Other causes of back pain

The symptoms of skeleto-muscular dysfunction in the back are sometimes mimicked by other illnesses not connected with the spine. One important reason why doctors have blood tests done in addition to X-rays is to eliminate the possibility that one of these illnesses is responsible for a patient's problem. The most serious of them is a tumour on the spine, causing back pain by compressing a nerve. This is no more than a remote possibility: in the great majority of cases the back pain is in fact found to be due to some mechanical disturbance.

Everyone is familiar with the ache in the bones that goes with influenza; many other viral infections are able to produce some degree of inflammation in the joints. Occasionally the pain may be particularly severe in the lower back. In such cases, however, there are sure to be other symptoms such as a high temperature or a sore throat, and if the infection affects the digestive organs, there may be diarrhoea, nausea and loss of appetite. These symptoms indicate that the back pain, which is part of the infection, is likely to go when the infection goes.

Kidney stones and kidney infections may also produce lower back pain, but there, too, there are usually tell-tale symptoms, such as fever and pain on passing urine.

Women

There are some kinds of non-spinal back pain that are reserved for women. Displacements of the womb, such as uterine prolapse, resulting from the strains of childbirth, can in some cases produce pain in the lower back. So can fibroids (benign tumours) in the womb. Both conditions can be put right, usually by surgical measures.

But normal conditions, such as pregnancy and menstruation, can also give rise to back pain. In pregnancy, hormonal changes before childbirth cause ligaments to soften and slacken, and this can cause strain, particularly in the sacroiliac joints; the weight of the growing foetus also throws additional strain on the spine. In menstruation, period cramps are sometimes felt as referred pain in the structures of the back.

Stress

The mental stress caused by an attack of back pain can reinforce the effects of muscle spasm, and in turn be made worse by it, in a vicious circle. Muscle spasm is a possible result of tension.

A major problem is fear of pain, sometimes not so much fear of the pain itself as fear that it is really more serious than anyone supposes. The remedy then is to seek authoritative reassurance.

It also seems very probable that mental tension, stress and anxiety, unexpressed fears and worries can actually start off an attack of backache by increasing muscular tension throughout the body. (This also makes you more vulnerable to muscular and joint strain which may even lead to some sort of mechanical displacement.) There are cases in which stress-reducing measures, or perhaps counselling, rather than treatment is what is needed to relieve the pain.

CHAPTER 6

WHERE DOES IT HURT?

THE body's central nervous system consists of the brain and the spinal cord, which is the brain's extension down the spinal canal. The nerve roots which pass in pairs out of the spinal cord at the level of each vertebra, and at the sacrum, proliferate into an abundant network of nerves, some as long as one metre, reaching to distant parts of the body. They carry information about injury along the spinal cord to the brain, which acts as a control centre, where the information is interpreted in the form of a sensation of pain. The sensory nerves which bring it are able to convey information about the type of injury; thus, the pain of a blow is different from that of a pinprick.

Pain is not sensed in the injured tissues themselves: the experience of pain is registered in the brain. For pain to be felt, there must be, or have been, a nerve supply. Some structures of the body have little, or none: for instance, the nucleus of an intervertebral disc. If it is damaged, no pain will be felt unless part of the disc presses on one of the nerve roots, the dural tube or on a ligament. Therefore the absence of pain does not necessarily mean that there has been no injury.

There can be an interval, sometimes days, between injury and sensation of pain. If you are concentrating hard on something else, you can often override the pain message. Sportsmen, in particular, often fail to realise that they have been hurt, until the game they are playing is over. A severe pain can mask a lesser pain, rather like a strong radio signal suppressing a weaker one. Thus it may not be until the more severe pain has responded to treatment that a secondary pain reveals the presence of a lesser injury.

Pain is both a mental and a physical event, and the extent to which it is found endurable depends largely on individual temperament. Some people give way rapidly, and take to their bed, while others grimly remain at their posts, regardless of suffering. There is an intelligent compromise between these extremes: an awareness that pain is, in general, a warning of injury or risk of injury through misuse or malfunction, which should not be neglected.

Referred pain

It is common for pain to be felt in an area much larger than the site of the injury, in remote tissues, which apparently have nothing wrong with them. This is called referred pain, and its mechanism is not well understood, but it probably occurs because the perception of pain can be felt as being anywhere in the network supplied by a particular nerve root. Information about any part of that region of the body reaches the brain along the same neural route. That is why people are able to feel pain in 'phantom' limbs that have been amputated. The pain message from the nerves in the stump are interpreted as if coming from a whole limb.

Pain in the back

Any of the tissues of the spine can be a source of pain except for the discs and the cartilage of the facet joints which have no nerve supply.

If the pain arises in the more superficial muscles, it can be identified as coming from a particular spot. Pain from around the facet joints and ligaments is less easy to pinpoint; and if it arises as the effect of a ruptured disc, it is felt too diffusely to locate precisely.

When it is the nerve root that is irritated, pain can be felt anywhere in the region which that nerve supplies. Thus, pain from injury to the sacral or lumbar nerve roots may be felt in the low back or to one side, or, very often, down one leg on the same side as the nerve. Disturbance to cervical or upper thoracic nerve roots may produce similar symptoms in an arm. Pain from the waist region is often felt in a buttock or groin. Similarly, pain originating in the ligaments and joints of the lumbar spine may be felt across the back of the hips, round the groin, across the buttocks, along the thigh to the knees or even further down the leg.

A sufferer's doctor or physiotherapist should be helped to identify the level in the spine of the source of pain by an exact description of where the pain is felt and its nature.

Root involvement; nerve root lesion

These are medical terms for the condition in which a nerve root is being irritated by being compressed or angulated, so that its blood supply is restricted. As well as pain, there may be other symptoms; if the nerve is of the motor type, whose function is to stimulate muscles into activity, the affected muscle may become weak, and have a reduced reflex response. It is seldom that all the nerves of a nerve root are damaged: as a rule, only a small proportion of them is affected.

Constant irritation of the nerve root in its dural sleeve may set up inflammation throughout the surrounding tissues, and this can cause adhesions to form between the walls of the spinal canal and the dural tube which sheathes the spinal cord, and also in the intervertebral foramina, the facet joints of the vertebrae, and the surrounding ligaments. These adhesions prevent the nerve root from moving easily in and out through its foramen with the normal movements of the spine and limbs, and this may cause pain. If a disc prolapses backwards, the prolapse can, depending on the size of the spinal canal, involve the cauda equina itself. This is rare, but if it happens, the resulting back and leg pain, with numbness, weakness and disturbance of bowel and bladder function, creates a surgical emergency.

Other symptoms

Pain may be accompanied by other symptoms, such as a feeling of dullness or heaviness, or perhaps coldness or a tingling sensation. When a lumbar nerve root is irritated or compressed, there may be weakened muscles as well as pain; a loss of sensitivity in the skin of the leg and the foot; pins and needles; tingling, heaviness, constriction or cramp.

When the spinal canal in the lumbar spine is constricted (spinal canal stenosis) so that there is pressure on the spinal cord, or when the bundle of nerve roots in the cauda equina is compressed, the symptoms, in addition to pain, may include weakness in the legs, so that walking becomes difficult, and weakness of the bladder and bowels, even incontinence, may result. Medical help should be sought without any delay.

CHAPTER 7

WHEN THE PAIN STRIKES

AN attack of back pain can take several forms. It may occur as a sudden, acute pain at a particular site, and be so severe that you cannot move; it may begin as a dull ache that becomes more severe during the following 24 hours; it may appear as a less painful sensation of stiffness in the muscles down one side of the body.

Back pain may follow a bout of unaccustomed exertion, such as clearing a garden path after a snowfall, or moving heavy furniture at spring cleaning. Or you may bend down awkwardly or with a sudden jerk, and feel that something has 'gone' in your back, but not experience really severe discomfort till the next morning, when inflammation will have built up in the damaged tissues. An attack may come on after a spell of mild, nagging backache which you had ignored in the hope that it would go away.

If you have had back trouble before, quite mild and accustomed exertion can cause it to recur; for example, reaching across the car from the driver's seat to open the passenger's door.

Immediate action

In the case of an acute attack of back pain, stop whatever you are doing, even if you are only sitting down.

Get to a bed, or some other level surface, and lie down. If you are locked in a stooped or sitting position and cannot straighten up, you may have to crawl, or, having reached the bed, may have to roll gently and slowly on to it.

Lying down takes the stress off your spine, so there should be less pain after a while. If your muscles are in spasm, this will help them to relax. You can then try to straighten yourself gradually, moving your legs gently, until your spine is straight, with its normal hollow in the small of the back. If you can achieve this, it may help to bring the attack to a speedier end.

If you have suffered an attack of back pain in the past and can tell that another is threatening, it may be wise to go and lie down straight away.

Which way to lie down?

The stress on the spine is least when you lie on your back, but this may not be the most comfortable (or, rather, least painful) position for you. There is no single 'correct' position, so lie on your side or stomach if this suits you better. The position you adopted during a previous attack may not be right for you now. (Lying on the floor, perhaps on a blanket or sleeping bag, is often more comfortable than a bed or sofa.)

You need not lie absolutely flat, but it is best to make do with only one pillow under your head.

Use whatever pillows or cushions you need to relieve strain. If lying on your back, a small pillow or folded towel in the small of the back and/or two or three pillows under the knees may make you more comfortable.

If you choose to lie on your side, try putting a pillow between you knees, to support the upper leg, and to prevent its weight from dragging on the spine and twisting it. The shoulders should be kept in line with the hips. Do not let the pelvis fall forward while the shoulders sink back against a pillow at the head. This would cause a definite torsion (twisting) in the spine, and you might feel worse stiffness and worse pain after spending some time in this position. Hugging a pillow in your arms may help to keep you lying correctly.

If your pain is in the vertebrae of the neck, you need something to give your neck support. Specially shaped neck pillows (which look rather like horse-collars) are available in department stores, but if you do not have one, roll up or twist a face towel lengthways, and wrap it round your neck. A soft pillow loosely tied in the centre and the filling shaken down to the two ends also makes a useful neck support. The thin middle part should lie behind the neck so the 'wings' support the side of the head.

Sitting, not lying

If there is nowhere for you to lie down – or if you feel more comfortable sitting down – try to find a suitable chair. It should have a firm seat, to support the pelvis evenly; a soft chair will allow the pelvis, together with the spine, to tilt sideways, causing uneven pressure and muscle spasm. The back rest should have a slight backward slope, with cushions between you and the back of the chair, so that you can recline; the pressure of your body weight will then not be taken by the vertebrae, but will be dispersed. Every part of the body should be supported, so that the muscles can relax completely.

The height of the seat should be such that the feet can rest flat on the floor without strain, or else they should be supported by a footstool.

Coping with the pain

Take a painkiller. Aspirin and ibuprofen may be specially effective where there is inflammation, but if you are allergic to either, take any painkiller that works for you. Do not be afraid of taking the full dosage recommended on the packet, for two or even three days at regular intervals, if necessary, with or after food (or at least a drink of milk). Do not try to use alcohol as a painkiller – especially not in combination with pain-killing drugs.

There are many commercial backache treatments on the market, and many people swear by some folk-remedy, perhaps one handed down in their family. Most of these 'cures' owe their reputation to the fact that, untreated or not, most back pain subsides in a few days. Any remedy being taken at the time usually gets the credit. There is probably no harm in using such treatments if you feel that they are doing you good, so long as they do not have untoward side-effects.

Hot and cold

Many people get relief from applying heat to the site of the pain. An ordinary rubber hot-water bottle inside a cover or wrapped in a towel is simple and effective, but make sure that it is not hotter than you can bear. You could also use an electric heating pad or a radiant lamp, but not too hot or for too long. Beware of burning yourself; sometimes pain in the back can reduce the sensitivity of the skin.

A hot bath may be comforting, but you may find getting into it – and, even more, getting out again – excessively painful. If you do have a bath, it is easier to kneel in order to get out, rather than from a sitting position. If there is a risk that you may get stuck, take your bath kneeling.

A gentle back rub can help to relieve back pain by encouraging muscles locked in spasm to relax, and by producing warmth through friction. Any willing member of your household can do it for you – making sure not to start with cold hands (the room should be warm, too). There is no advantage in using ointment or liniment, but no harm in doing so.

For those who can bear it, the application of cold can also be effective in relieving pain, by numbing its site. If you have no ice-bag, you can use a hot-water bottle or even a polythene bag filled with crushed ice-cubes, or a pack of frozen peas will do very well. Make sure there is a damp towel between the ice and the skin. This treatment, like the heat one, should only be used in moderation (and only if found effective). Ten to twenty minutes is usual, or up to half an hour, but you should be aware that ice can 'burn' if the application is too prolonged. Anyone with a heart condition should avoid this form of self-help.

You may find that the pain is worse on the second day, and that it hurts to cough or sneeze. You will probably not need to be told to lie as still as you can, to avoid pain. Getting out of bed will be difficult and unpleasant, and to be attempted only in order to go to the lavatory (men may find a bed-bottle helpful).

Calling your doctor?

When the pain first strikes, it can be frightening, and your first impulse may be to call your GP. But if the pain is only in your back, there is no need to be precipitate – and certainly no need to get your doctor out of bed. The pain should become less acute in a day or two, and the whole episode will probably last three or four days, which you should spend in bed, if possible – you may not feel able to do anything else. If you do call your doctor right away, the chances are that he will tell you to stay in bed, take painkillers, and ring again in two or three days' time if the pain has not become easier.

But if you have any other signs and symptoms, such as numbness, pins and needles, tingling; if you pass water very frequently, or have trouble doing so; if you experience weakness, giddiness or nausea; if you have severe referred pain (that is, somewhere else, as well as in the back), do consult your doctor right away.

Staying in bed

'Put a board under your mattress' is the piece of advice that the back pain victim hears from practically everybody. But this should be necessary only if your bed has a very soft base or an old, sagging mattress. There is no need to support a reasonably firm mattress. However, if you do need a bed board but have not got one, ask someone to drag your mattress on to the floor. Or simply do what many back sufferers do, sleep on a quilt or sleeping bag spread on the floor itself, using pillows, as already described, to relieve pressure and to keep your spine straight. When in acute pain, it is difficult to get down on to the floor and even harder to get up again; going via the kneeling position helps.

If you lie mostly on your back, you may find it most comfortable to support your legs, from the knees down, on a pile of cushions; or on a chair or a stool or pouffe if you are sleeping on the floor. In this position, the back is kept from arching by being pressed firmly against the mattress (or floor).

If you have managed to find a comfortable position, the tendency is to stay put, but you should try to vary it from time to time, for the good of your circulation. Also, if you remain immobile because of back pain you may find yourself feeling stiff all over after a time. Changing position may call for some courage: do it slowly and gradually. Changing from a horizontal to a vertical position is what hurts most, so do not try to sit up. As for turning over in bed, you may find this easier to do if you bend your knees, bringing your heels up towards your buttocks, and, keeping your shoulder in line with your hips, let the knees fall to one side and use the weight of your legs to roll you over.

For getting out of bed, try this method: turn on your side, then edge over to the side of the bed, keeping your knees bent; then let your legs slide over the edge, acting as a counterweight as you push yourself upright with your arms. Have a chair at hand to lean on as you get to your feet.

In the end, you will probably work out for yourself, by painful trial and error, the method of getting out of bed that causes the least discomfort. Even so, try to limit the number of occasions of doing it, especially during the first day or so. Moderation in eating and drinking will limit the number of times you have to go to the lavatory; and you may not have much appetite in any case. Avoid alcohol, which may interact with the painkilling drugs you are taking; some people find that it makes the pain worse.

You may find yourself temporarily constipated, which may be the effect of taking some types of painkiller, or of immobility, or fear of the pain that getting out of bed causes. This is a temporary problem, and there is no need to worry or do anything about it.

Keeping moving

At this stage you cannot do much in the way of exercise, but try to move your legs at regular intervals. The longer you remain immobile, the longer it will take you to recover your strength and mobility.

Even when you are suffering severe pain, and are frightened to move, there are bound to be some movements you can make without pain.

Start with these. Try wriggling your toes, bending and circling your ankles, working the feet up and down, bending and extending the knees. Do this for a few minutes, every hour or so. If any movement causes you pain, avoid it, and try to find another that does not. In between spells of leg movements, do some slow deep breathing.

A weight off your mind

It may not be easy for you to induce your tensed muscles to relax if at the same time you are brooding about the work and other obligations for which you are now temporarily disabled. A serene frame of mind may seem rather too much to expect from someone who is being racked by acute back pain, but relaxation involves both body and mind, so if you can find a way of relaxing your mental tension, the pain may affect you less.

The best thing to do is to accept the situation, and abandon, as much as possible, feelings of guilt about neglected work, missed appointments and so on. You are a victim of *force majeure*: the matter is out of your hands for the time being. You will have to ask someone to do some telephoning for you, cancelling engagements, and arranging for other people to stand in for you, at home and at work. Accept the need to rest and look after yourself for a few days. To not be tempted to get up too soon. The more you can allow yourself to be philosophical about the situation, the more rapid is recovery likely to be. For a while the world will have to roll on its course without you. This advice is more easily given than followed.

But don't become an invalid

Other people can affect your back pain. Some families enjoy making a fuss of an invalid and that may actually inhibit the natural desire to resume normal life. One danger with giving in to back pain for too long is the stiffness and weakness which ensue.

Supporters of the 'pain confrontation' school of thought argue that there is no evidence that activity is harmful and that, contrary to common belief, it does not necessarily even aggravate the pain as long as specific activities which increase the load on the spine are avoided. Increased activity may promote bone and muscle strength and may increase endorphin (pain reducing hormone) levels and reduce sensitivity to pain. They also claim that there is no evidence that early return to work increases the likelihood of future recurrences. These views are not universally accepted.

Proper controlled trials have yet to be carried out to determine which treatments are most effective for various types of back pain, so that a rational basis can be developed for choosing the most effective treatment for individual patients.

When the pain starts to go

Most episodes of acute back pain grow less severe within two or three days, when the sufferer can start to get up and about again. On the first day this should be for only a couple of hours at a time, with spells of rest in between, increasing gradually on succeeding days.

Getting dressed may be difficult, especially putting on socks, shoes, tights and trousers, and it may be wisest to stay in dressing gown and slippers for the first day or so you are up. If you feel that you must get dressed, wear whatever is easiest to put on. A woman can choose a dress rather than trousers, and leave off tights. Slip-on shoes are preferable to lace-ups. A long-handled shoe horn can be a help.

If you must put on tights or trousers, put them on while lying on your back with your knees bent; but do not raise your hips to

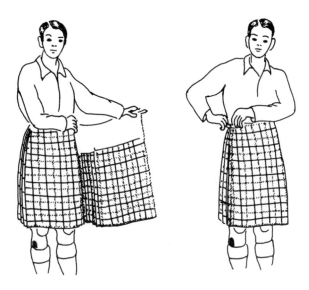

Highlanders have no problem! The kilt just wraps round; so the back can be kept quite straight

pull them right up, which could arch your spine – get off the bed and then do the pulling-up.

There is a gentle exercise that is worth trying when you are feeling less sore. If the pain is in the lower back, while standing put the palms of your hands on your hips, on the bony crests on either side of the pelvis, and holding it steady, sway your shoulders backwards beyond the level of your hips, thus extending the vertebral column. Do this slowly and gently, and stop at once if the pain increases.

If the pain is in the upper part of the back, interlock your fingers behind your head; press your elbows back in line with the shoulder joints, pulling the shoulder-blades together. Press your head slowly and gently against the fingers, while pressing your hands forwards and up, thus applying a mild traction force to the neck. Again, stop if the pain increases.

Do not drive a car, and take care, when you are a passenger, how you get into your seat. Bending at neck or waist may bring the pain on again. Get in slowly, preferably by standing with your back to the seat, then sitting down with your legs outside, and then slowly swivelling round while lifting your legs in, with your hands behind the thigh.

Until you are completely fit again, do your best to avoid lifting and carrying heavy weights. If you really must carry things – essential shopping, for instance, divide the load equally in two, one bag in each hand. Or you could try a back pack, which someone else would have to put on for you. Above all, make sure not to repeat the movement which brought on the attack, if you know which one it was; and in general, avoid twisting and bending movements.

If the pain does not go

If by the third day the pain is as bad as ever, it is time to see the doctor. If you are unable to get into a car, or have nobody to drive you, it will have to be a home visit. The doctor may ask:

- about the nature of the pain – you should tell him whether it is a sharp or stabbing or burning pain, or a dull ache; whether you feel it at one side or radiating to other places, the arms or legs, for instance; whether you are having tingling sensations there, or a feeling of numbness;

- about the origin of the pain – tell him when and where you first felt it; whether any particular activity had brought it on; whether it started suddenly or developed gradually; whether there are any postures or movements which make it worse – or better;

- about the duration of the pain – tell him how long it is since it started; whether you have it all the time; whether it has got worse since the onset, or stayed the same; whether there are times during the day or night when you feel it more.

The doctor may not follow this pattern; listen carefully to the questions and be as precise as you can in your answers. The doctor may also ask you about the kind of work you do – active or sedentary, domestic or outdoor – in order to assess the stresses that it may exert on your spine.

The physical examination
You will be asked to remove your outer clothes. The doctor will ask you to do a number of things to enable him to assess your problem.

While standing upright, you will be asked to bend, as well as you can, backwards, forwards and sideways, so that the doctor can see which of these movements causes you most discomfort. This gives him a clue as to which of the joints or muscles of the back may be involved.

As you lie prone (face downwards) on the couch, the doctor will palpate, that is, explore by finger pressure, the tender area of your back, as well as other areas where you may not have felt pain before, but which are now found to hurt when prodded. This is because when the source of the pain is a nerve root, the pain may be felt all along the nerve.

As you lie supine (on your back) on the couch, the doctor will raise each of your legs in turn, with the knee straight. This stretches the sciatic nerve, and he wants to see how far he can do this without aggravating the pain.

The doctor may try other movements, to find out whether certain nerves are working properly. He will check whether there is any loss of sensation in any part of your body, and whether your reflexes are normal.

In most cases, back pain is due to a dysfunction of the spine. However, there may be other causes, which the doctor is bound to consider: for instance, kidney disease, or a peptic ulcer. So the doctor will probably examine your abdomen as well. In women, backache may be caused by gynaecological trouble, such as fibroids or a prolapse of the womb (but such a cause is not at all common); however, low backache from any cause may be worse before a menstrual period.

If the doctor suspects that a cause of your pain is a degenerated or prolapsed disc, he will probably tell you to return to bed, because rest is essential to permit any inflammation to subside, or to allow the disc bulge to shrink somewhat, thus releasing the pressure on the nerve that is causing the pain.

The doctor may give you painkillers, possibly by injection, and also tablets to take at home. He may also prescribe a tranquilliser, not to stop you worrying, but because of the beneficial effect of a relaxed mood on muscles in spasm. Tell the doctor if you happen to know that any of these remedies upsets you.

The doctor may propose treatment by a physiotherapist; if you want to go and see an osteopath, the doctor may refer you to one with medical qualifications (but there is no need for a GP's referral in order to see any osteopath of your choice. An advantage for someone with acute back pain is that the osteopath may be able to see him/her promptly – but treatment outside the National Health Service is expensive). Or the GP may refer you to a hospital out-patient clinic for a specialist examination.

CHAPTER 8

SPECIALIST EXAMINATION

IF your back trouble is not better after a few weeks, or, having got better, keeps recurring, or your GP thinks there could be some uncommon reason for your trouble, he may suggest that you should be seen by a specialist. Usually this means going to a hospital as an out-patient (or being admitted as an in-patient for a day, for investigation) to attend a consultant's clinic in the orthopaedic or rheumatology or neurology department. The out-patient appointment may be for a date weeks or even months ahead, though if your case is considered urgent on medical grounds, you may be seen more quickly.

In his letter of referral, your GP will give the specialist a history of your trouble, mentioning his own conclusions from the examination he gave you and any tests he has had carried out, such as X-rays.

The specialist's aim will be twofold: to exclude the possibility that the pain is caused by disease in some other organ, and to find out its origin and cause. The questions he asks, the examination he carries out and any further investigations he orders will all be directed to this purpose, their scope depending on whether this is your first spell of back trouble, or a recurrent problem which has not yielded to treatment.

He will want to know about your previous medical history, operations, severe injuries or prolonged illnesses, and whether you are currently having treatment for any other condition.

When he has completed his tests and investigations, he may be in a position to tell you whether there is any serious disease. If he does not reassure you on this point, do not hesitate to ask him.

Questions and answers

The first thing the specialist will ask is where the pain and other symptoms are, and how far they extend. Try to point them out as clearly as possible. Be prepared to go into considerable detail, if asked. He will want to know how long ago the trouble began; what you were doing when it started (or just before); what the symptoms were like to start with, and how they have changed since. In other words, whether you are between attacks, in continuous pain, getting better or worse.

If by the time you see the specialist your back is better, say so. Specialists are used to this, and he will not think that his time has been wasted. His job is to get you completely well, and to prevent further trouble.

You should tell the specialist what makes the pain better, and what makes it worse – things like bending, sitting, walking and so forth – and the effect the pain has on your usual activities. Tell him about your state of mind, too. If you are under any strain in your work, home, relationships or other personal factors, tell him, in case it has any bearing on your back pain. The severity and unpredictable nature of the pain, and the disruption it is bound to have caused to your daily life, may be affecting you emotionally.

It may be difficult to describe symptoms other than pain, such as heaviness, dullness, tightness, numbness and weakness. Numbness, for example, means different things to different people. Some use it in a general way to describe a sensation that a leg, for instance, has 'gone to sleep'. But it may also mean, more precisely, that the skin itself has lost all sensation and that you could scald it without feeling pain. Weakness, for instance, could describe feeling limp because of pain, or else being forced to drag your toes along because you cannot bend up your ankle. Analyze the feeling or pain carefully, explain it as descriptively as you can and try to make sure that the doctor understands what you are trying to describe. It is important for the patient to tell the doctor what he feels, not what he thinks he ought to feel. Spontaneity is the patient's great asset. Analysis is the doctor's job.

It is useful to be able to give information about any previous back trouble before the current attack. But when it is a long and complex story, it may be difficult to know how much to tell your doctor. On the whole, unless asked directly, it is better to avoid recounting in detail what has been said to you by various doctors, surgeons, chiropractors and physiotherapists you may have seen in the past. Doctors like to make their own diagnosis and it does not really help to give them other people's. The important thing is where the pain was and whether you had to go to bed or could continue at work; how many times you have had the pain since and whether the pain then, and subsequently, was like it is now; what investigations were made (if you know); whether you have had any treatment and, if so, what helped and what made it worse.

Going to a specialist can be an intimidating occasion. You may feel more confident if you jot down some notes beforehand, with dates, of your case history so that you do not return home wishing you had mentioned all sorts of things you forgot at the time.

Physical examination

Be prepared to strip down to (bra and) pants with socks or tights off. The spine will have to be examined and the examination is bound to hurt a bit, because your pain is the focus of interest. Be as accurate as you can about what you feel while the doctor is examining you.

The order and extent of the doctor's examination may vary but usually it begins by an inspection of the posture of your spine, because this can be affected both by your present symptoms and by some deformity.

The range of movements you can make, and the way you make them are looked at while you bend forwards, sideways and backwards; some hospitals have a special device for measuring this. The doctor moves your neck, arms and legs, to test for signs of increased tension in the nerve roots, and also tests muscle strength in the back, abdomen, arms and legs.

Your spine is felt for signs of tenderness, muscle spasm or deformity. The sensitivity of the skin on the arms and hands or the foot, leg, thigh and buttock is checked by touch and pin-pricks. Your reflexes are tested at the elbow, wrist, ankle, knee and sole of the foot.

X-rays

You will almost certainly be sent to the X-ray department, either there and then, or at a later appointment, to have X-rays (radiographs) taken of your spine.

If you are a woman of childbearing age, you should first be asked about the date of your last menstrual period. There is a 'ten-day rule' allowing X-rays to be taken only during the ten days after the start of a menstrual period, before the probable time of ovulation. Later than this, there exists a possibility of conception, and an embryo could be damaged by irradiation.

Generally, three or four views of the spine are taken. Sometimes, one sideways view is taken with the spine bent fully forwards and another with it arched backwards. This can be uncomfortable, but do your best to relax and keep still so that the picture is not blurred. It is done like this in order to assess movement between these two postures at each vertebral level – whether it is absent or excessive, or abnormal in some other way. One film may be taken in the standing position because the alignment of the bones and disc spaces may be significantly different when they are weight-bearing from when you are lying down.

On the film, the shadows of the bones show up in excellent detail, particularly if you are slim. It is possible to assess the size and shape of the spinal canal and its exits, which may be relevant. The discs themselves do not show, only the spaces they occupy. (Remember this in case you get a chance to look at your own X-rays.)

The X-rays are seen by the consultant, and may also be seen by the radiologist – a doctor specialising in X-ray diagnosis.

X-rays can reveal a fractured or cracked vertebra, or show the presence of degenerative changes in the vertebrae, such as the formation of osteophytes, or of bone thickening, as well as signs of abnormalities such as misalignment of vertebrae, of deformities and potential mechanical weaknesses.

X-rays can, however, be deceptive and show up an abnormality which causes the person no pain or, where a person is obviously in great pain, the X-rays may reveal nothing. The doctor may well not find anything abnormal, even though the patient may be suffering from acute disc prolapse, or serious muscular injury, because discs, muscles, ligaments and other 'soft' tissues are not radio-opaque: they do not show up on X-rays, or only very faintly. If the space occupied by a disc is seen to be reduced, it suggests that the disc has been flattened, but this does not necessarily indicate a prolapse.

Further tests

Depending on what has been learned so far, and on your symptoms, further tests may be carried out. In most cases, however, it is unlikely that they will have to be done; at any rate, not all of them.

Most surgeons insist on some such investigation before deciding whether to recommend an operation. Some of these tests may require you to be admitted to hospital for a couple of days.

Myelography or radiculography

This is a method of making the dural tube show up in X-rays, by injecting a contrast medium – a radio-opaque liquid – into the cerebro-spinal fluid around the spinal cord. This is done under local anaesthesia, by lumbar puncture, the needle being inserted through the skin of the back between a pair of vertebrae at the appropriate level.

Using an image-intensifying screen, the radiologist can see whether the spinal canal is abnormally narrow and whether anything is obstructing it – such as the bulge of a prolapsed disc, or a degenerated joint. These show up as an indentation on the dural tube, or an obliteration of part of a dural root sleeve. In rare cases, back pain may be caused by a tumour on the spinal cord, and this, too, would be shown up by myelography. As a matter of routine, a sample of the cerebro-spinal fluid is taken for laboratory testing.

The lumbar puncture is done while you lie on a table which can be raised to the vertical, so that the radiologist can observe the movement of the contrast medium in the dural tube as you are tilted up and down. The table may also tilt sideways, or the apparatus rotate in relation to the table, so that the radiologist can view the spine from different angles. He will probably take still radiographs to record the significant findings. Most of the time, however, he will be studying the picture on a television monitor which you may be able to see, too.

When the myelography is finished, you may be sent to a ward, with instructions to rest quietly for up to 24 hours and may be warned of the possibility of getting severe headache or nausea for a while, as an after-effect. Myelography is, to say the least, uncomfortable. Nowadays, a water-based contrast medium is used. This is soon eliminated by the body, and does not usually cause irritation in the tissues of the spine.

Discography

This is a similar procedure, used for making discs visible on X-rays, and may show up prolapse bulges that do not show up on myelograms. The contrast medium is injected into the centre of discs, usually the three lowest lumbar discs. Only a small quantity of contrast medium is used, and the patient does not have to be tipped about. In a healthy disc, the medium stays discretely in the middle, but in a degenerated one it spreads out and may show the extent and direction of any prolapse.

There are some other radiological investigations for someone with severe symptoms or repeated attacks (these investigations are the exception rather than the rule for uncomplicated cases of back and sciatic pain). For example, the nerve root itself can be injected outside the spinal canal – *extraspinal radiculography*. The epidural space can be injected via the gap between the bones of the sacrum and coccyx to show the space in the spinal canal surrounding the dural tube – *epidurography*. Alternatively, the medium can be injected direct into the bone of the spinous process and then drains into the veins of the epidural space – *epidural venography*. More commonly, this is done by inserting a catheter in the femoral vein in the groin and then injecting the lumbar veins – *ascending lumbar venography*. In *stereoradiography*, X-rays are taken to give a three-dimensional effect.

CAT (or CT) scanning

This stands for *computerised-axial tomography*, a new technique not yet available everywhere. It can be used on any part of the body, but is particularly useful for examining delicate and not easily accessible tissues, such as the brain and the spinal canal.

It takes rather longer than ordinary X-rays, but is not unpleasant. You have to lie still on a sort of couch for 15 to 20 minutes while X-rays are taken all round the spine, and a computer combines the information they give to produce a series of pictures of a cross-section of the spine at any given point, and also of the adjacent tissues. CAT-scanning uses lower dosages of radiation than other X-ray techniques. The technique is sensitive enough to show up disc bulges and degeneration even without a contrast medium, though it can also be combined with myelography.

Ultrasound scanning
This painless technique works rather like radar: by means of a microphone-like probe, which is passed over the back, inaudible ultrasound waves are directed at the spine, and the echoes which are bounced back are picked up by the probe. They are used to build up a picture of the spine on a monitor screen; one use of ultrasound is to measure the width of the spinal canal.

Magnetic resonance imaging (MR or MRI)
This is still largely a research tool, but is available at some hospitals for use in diagnosis. It is very helpful in diagnosing disc prolapse because it shows fluid/solid interfaces very clearly. It can demonstrate epidural fat, root sleeves, nerve roots and the vertebral canal, neural foramina and facet joints. It is particularly useful for examining the brain and spinal cord and may, eventually, become the preferred method of investigation for neck disc problems. It does not use X-rays but a powerful magnetic field to observe and measure 'spins' of atomic nuclei. At present, there are no known risks to the technique, but it cannot be used if you have any metal artificial joints, plates etc., so you would have to tell the doctor or radiographer about them.

Electromyography (EMG)
This is done in some hospitals if damage to the nerve root is suspected. The functioning of the nerves which supply muscles is tested by using an apparatus for amplifying and recording the electrical activity produced in the muscles. A fine needle electrode is inserted into the muscles of the legs – sometimes those of the

back also; this is usually not very painful, not more than an ordinary injection, and leaves no side-effects.

The doctor may, in addition, do other tests to measure the speed with which nerves conduct the impulses in response to stimulation.

Blood tests

A blood sample may be taken, by means of a hypodermic syringe, from a vein in the arm, and sent to the haematological laboratory for tests, in order to obtain more general medical information, particularly about the possibility of inflammatory joint disease, anaemia, viral infection, cancer.

CHAPTER 9

TREATMENT

OVER the centuries, victims of back pain have submitted to a vast variety of treatments. The bizarre nature of some of these testifies to the sufferers' desperation: they were willing to try anything – even, it is said, having a tame bear tread on their back. In spite of great advances in medical science generally, these unorthodox treatments – except, perhaps, the bear – are still in with a chance.

Back pain therapy presents special problems. It is often difficult to diagnose accurately the cause of an attack of back pain. Damage to the structures of the back does not, as a rule, show on the surface, many do not show up on X-ray and even in-depth specialist investigations may not reveal anything obviously amiss.

Moreover, very often back pain is out of proportion to the problem causing it; although the pain is severe and disabling, the structural damage may be minor, and one accepted view is that it will heal, given time, with or without treatment. Another school of thought considers this to be shortsighted and holds that correct treatment by a qualified therapist will expedite recovery and may help to break down scar tissue, the presence of which can produce long-term problems.

If any treatment is given, it is sure to get the credit for the recovery. But the next time it is tried on someone, it may not work, either because it is valueless, or because the problem is not the same – it is hard to say which.

The information gleaned from each case may be of only limited use in the next one, and the treatment of back pain has had to be largely empirical. The fact that diagnoses are often less than accurate makes the choice of therapy problematic and specific therapies which exist for one condition are sometimes applied erroneously to another. There is no scientific body of knowledge which allows a doctor or any other practitioner to state with certainty that a particular treatment will cure the trouble.

The rationale of advising rest, and particularly bed rest, is based on the clinical observation that lying down may relieve pain. This applies to a diagnosis of disc prolapse: intradiscal pressure is lowest in the lying position. However, disc prolapse constitutes only a small percentage of all low-back pain and treatment for disc prolapse cannot necessarily be extrapolated to all low-back pain. This undermines the time-honoured belief that bed-rest is the first line of treatment for acute attacks of back pain.

Basically, however, the treatment which is currently offered by most doctors starts with conservative methods.

Conservative treatment

The most obvious way of coping with back pain is avoiding the postures and movements that cause it, or make it worse. It is based on the supposition that, where there is no serious disease, the problem will diminish if what aggravates it is removed. The treatment consists of avoiding activity: not going to work, avoiding painful chores, staying in bed if necessary. It is better to avoid a painful movement than to take painkillers to allow you to make the movement.

Painkillers
The most frequently employed analgesics are aspirins in various forms, paracetamol, also mixtures of these and other drugs such as codeine phosphate which are all available without prescription; also ibuprofen (sold under the name of Nurofen) which is a non-steroid anti-inflammatory drug. For more intractable pain, the doctor may prescribe other painkillers which you cannot buy over the counter.

Muscle relaxants are another line of approach. They are intended to relax the back muscles which tend to be held tense to the point of spasm, when there is pain, so making the pain worse.

Some relaxant drugs are addictive and are likely to be prescribed for only a short period. The doctor may also prescribe anti-inflammatory drugs. Sleeping pills are sometimes prescribed for people whose back pain prevents sleep, if a painkiller on its own is not sufficient.

None of these drugs acts directly on the source of the trouble to cure it. They only make you more comfortable and so relax the muscles while natural repair or restoration of normal alignment takes place.

Side-effects

Any pill or combination of pills prescribed for you may have side-effects. Few medicines are without them. Often the side-effect is minor – for instance, a dry mouth. Many of these drugs tend to constipate, which will not matter if it is only for a few days; others may upset the stomach or make you dizzy or fuddled, and that could be worse than the backache. Some people are allergic to aspirin, and may also react to ibuprofen.

There are standard doses for all these pills, but some people need either more or less than the usual to produce the desired effect. If a drug does not work for you or if the unpleasantness of the side-effect is greater than the benefit, you should stop taking the drug and report what has happened to the doctor. He may prescribe an alternative for you.

Injection therapy

In some cases, pain can be relieved by injecting pain-relieving drugs directly into the area of the spine where the pain appears to be localised. It can be effective for treating 'trigger points' (fibrositis), small, very painful nodules of muscle often in the buttocks, neck and shoulders, pressure on which spreads the pain over a wide area.

Usually a corticosteroid drug is injected, together with a local anaesthetic. The relief may not be immediate, or long-lasting, and a number of injections may be required for the treatment to be effective.

Some doctors inject into a strained ligament a sclerosing – that is, thickening – agent, to encourage the production of fibrous tissue, of which ligaments are made. This may encourage them to become thicker and stronger, but it is not certain that this is how sclerosant injections work.

Epidural injections are used for pain which has not yielded to any other methods. These injections are given into the epidural space between the dural tube and the spinal canal, at the lower end of the sacrum. They consist of a corticosteroid drug mixed with a local anaesthetic. This numbs the tube, and reduces inflammation, such as that set up by a prolapsed disc. The injection cannot put right the prolapse itself, but in most cases time is the best healer for this, and epidural injections, like other pain-relieving measures, make the period of waiting seem less interminable.

Much backache arises from the facet joints rather than from disc protrusion. Pain originating in facet joints can radiate down the leg and mimic sciatica. In some cases, injecting steroids and a local anaesthetic into the joint can stop the pain. If relief is only temporary, the nerve to the facet can be destroyed, producing permanent relief. The technique is one which is reserved for experts, usually anaesthetists running a pain clinic.

Chemonucleolysis (discolysis)

This method of treating a prolapsed disc is being offered in a few centres in Britain. It is a chemical alternative to disc surgery, and is used when time and rest have failed to reduce a disc protrusion which is involving a sciatic nerve. It has much the same success rate as surgery, with different but no fewer risks, and perhaps less discomfort and less disablement during the recovery period.

'Lysis' means dissolution. In chemonucleolysis, an enzyme called chymopapain is injected into the centre of the damaged disc nucleus. This enzyme is derived from the papaya (pawpaw) fruit (and is used also as a meat tenderiser). It has the effect of dissolving the more complex proteins in the nucleus and in the prolapsed part of the disc. Afterwards, the disc shrinks, becoming perceptibly narrower and stiffer. Because of this reduction in volume, the compression of the nerve is relaxed.

Chemonucleolysis is most successful in young people, and where the disc prolapse is fairly recent and has not had time to cause nerve damage or to produce adhesions. It is least successful in the case of extruded disc material having broken away completely – because the chymopapain cannot reach it.

How it is done
Chemonucleolysis is done under sedation or local anaesthesia; X-rays are used to place the needle accurately through the skin of the back. The orthopaedic surgeon or neurosurgeon first injects some contrast medium into the disc to assess the damage; then, with the needle still in place, injects chymopapain. If the treatment is successful, the sciatic pain in the leg goes, sometimes with dramatic rapidity; however, most patients have some back ache for a week or two.

There is a considerable risk if the chymopapain is injected in the wrong place, it is a technique only for experts. Even then, there is a small risk of an allergic reaction to chymopapain in patients who have become sensitised to it through eating tenderised meat, or who are allergic to papaya. Drugs are usually administered before the treatment, to minimise the risk of this.

Corsets and other supports

For supporting the different levels of the spine there exist various devices, such as corsets, belts and collars. Even though these supports are restrictive and cumbersome, many people with back trouble are ready to put up with them, for the sake of the benefits they bring.

They slow down all activity, and restrain many small movements of muscles, so helping muscular spasm to relax. Supports also prevent pain to some extent, by keeping the wearer from extremes of movement. A corset can help with acute pain and when an activity that might bring on pain cannot be avoided – housework, for instance.

Corsets are probably helpful in acute attacks and in the early stages of recovery. They should, however, not be considered as a long-term measure, because they have a tendency to weaken the muscles, and create a dependency on them (making the wearer believe that he cannot do without the corset). It is seldom necessary to continue with a corset for a long period; this should only be done after a positive decision by a specialist.

Lumbar corsets and belts also act to encourage correct lifting and bending; being unable to bend at the waist, the wearer has to lift things by bending, correctly, at the knees. They increase the intra–abdominal pressure which protects the spine in lifting actions by spreading the load, so that it bears less heavily on the lumbar joints.

Cervical collars are sometimes prescribed for neck injuries, or in the case of degenerated neck vertebrae. They work in a similar way to corsets, giving support and preventing inappropriate movement. With the rigid sort, the wearer can neither nod nor shake his head. The soft kind of cervical collar is often worn at night only, to support the neck during sleep.

How to obtain a corset

The National Health Service supplies many different types of spinal and abdominal supports. Usually it is the consultant at the hospital or clinic who prescribes one, but in some areas the GP can do so, via the physiotherapy department. Corsets should be properly fitted by a physiotherapist or other professional health worker. They can be bought privately but they are very expensive. Ordering one by mail order may be unsatisfactory or uncomfortable because it may not fit you.

For an acute attack, you may be supplied with an 'instant' corset – that is, one that is handed to you in the out-patients' clinic, so that you do not have to wait to have one made to measure. It comes in a few standard sizes, and is fastened either with buckles or with Velcro, so that it can be pulled tight around the hips and the lower back. Some lumbar supports and cervical collars are made in the occupational therapy or, more likely, the physiotherapy department, and may be made in one day, while you wait.

After a spinal operation, you may be prescribed a tailored fabric corset or other support. General hospitals arrange for corsets to be made by surgical appliance manufacturers, but some orthopaedic hospitals have their own appliance departments. The fitter is responsible to the consultant for the correct making, fitting and function. The consultant can arrange for a corset to be altered.

A corset does not necessarily have to be worn all the time. You should ask for specific instructions about when and for how long you should wear yours. Talc on the skin underneath the corset reduces friction and may make wearing it more comfortable.

CHAPTER 10

PHYSIOTHERAPY

BACK pain frequently responds well to physiotherapy, the treatment by physical methods, as an alternative or adjunct to drugs or surgery. The methods include several different therapies, manipulative procedures, therapeutic movement or exercises, treatment with heat, cold and with electrical equipment. The aim is to help restore the function of the body and rehabilitate the patient: it also includes advice and instruction on posture and daily activities.

The profession

Training for a physiotherapist in this country is a three- or four-year course at one of the schools of physiotherapy attached to hospitals or to a polytechnic or university. A student who passes the examinations qualifies for membership of the Chartered Society of Physiotherapy and therefore for state registration. Only state-registered physiotherapists can work within the National Health Service. Physiotherapists work in hospitals, in local authority clinics, in the community, in special schools, in industry and sports, and also in private practice (and may visit a patient in his own home). It is not a closed profession (anyone can put up a plate and set up in practice as a physiotherapist), but only those who have passed the examinations recognised by the Chartered Society of Physiotherapy can put MCSP after their name; and those who are state-registered, can put SRP. Contact the Chartered Society of Physiotherapy at 14 Bedford Row, London WC1R 4ED (tel: 071-242 1941).

Although physiotherapy is an independent profession and practitioners may accept people for treatment who are not referred by doctors, physiotherapists usually require patients to be referred to them by a doctor, for professional and legal reasons. It is possible to go directly to a physiotherapist, who will probably then contact the patient's GP.

There are chartered physiotherapists in private practice. They may be able to give treatment more quickly than through the NHS.

All health authorities have physiotherapy services. Patients are referred to them, often by the consultant at the out-patient clinic they are attending. In many cases, physiotherapy clinics will accept patients by direct referral from GPs.

The doctor making the referral sends to the physiotherapy clinic the necessary information about the patient and the condition, including X-ray photographs, with suggestions for the aims of the treatment, but leaving the choice of treatment to the physiotherapist's discretion. All physiotherapists assess their patients and plan out the treatment programme.

The treatment

More than one method of treatment may be tried; each patient's condition and progress is reassessed regularly, and the treatment altered accordingly. For example, a patient with very acute back pain may initially be given heat treatment and an instant support to wear. This may be followed after a couple of days by traction or gentle mobilisation, and possibly later by a vigorous manipulation, and the treatment usually includes a regimen of exercises and instruction on how to lift and move safely.

What a patient does when not having treatment plays an important role in recovery; the physiotherapist will, therefore, usually advise what he should do between treatments. Patients who hope and expect that the physiotherapist will work on them to get them better are not pleased to discover that they are, instead, expected to participate actively.

Manipulative procedures

This is the term covering a very wide range of techniques from the very gentle to the more vigorous.

Soft tissue techniques

The most familiar soft tissue technique is massage whereby muscles, tendons and ligaments are mobilised by the therapist's hands and fingers in order to induce relaxation, increase local circulation and movement and relieve pain. Massage is usually used in conjunction with other procedures.

Regional mobilisation

For people with spinal problems, this is used to treat areas of stiffness and altered movement accompanied by pain. The techniques which are used often have an effect on groups of joints and their surrounding tissues. Regional mobilisation involves gentle and repeated passive movement of the affected area to relieve pain and increase the range of movement.

Localised mobilisation

When pain arises from a spinal disorder, the physiotherapist locates the level of the spine producing the symptoms, and may then use localised mobilisation techniques to relieve the pain and restore the normal range of movement. Localised mobilisations consist of passive, small-range, repetitive movements.

The most vigorous of the manipulative procedures is the application of a deliberate thrust to increase joint mobility, taking the movement a little farther than it goes in ordinary active movements, but within the normal passive range.

Traction

This is a longitudinal stretching force applied along the axis of the tissues and is a form of regional mobilisation. It has been known for centuries that back pain can sometimes be relieved in this way. It is not known, however, why traction works when it does. Some practitioners have claimed that pulling the vertebral bodies slightly apart eases the pressure on a prolapsed disc. But this in itself would not make the extruded disc material shrink back, nor repair the ruptured outer casing. One theory was that the vacuum produced in the intervertebral space would withdraw the extruded disc material away from the nerve, but bioengineering experiments have now shown this to be unlikely. Studies have suggested that the amount of traction necessary to achieve actual separation of vertebral bodies is far greater than that ever applied by way of pelvic traction in a physiotherapy department. Possibly traction works by reducing tension or spasm in the back and hip muscles, or by easing the strain on the facet joints. There is no conclusive evidence. Many people have found relief in this way, but if you are one of the people for whom it does not work, there is no point in persisting with it.

There are several ways of applying traction involving, in many cases, the use of special apparatus. The magnitude of the pulling force, the position in which it is given and the time for which it is applied will determine the effects of the traction. If the traction makes the pain worse at the time, the treatment is stopped. If the pain is worse after traction, the treatment should be discontinued. Patients with severe back pain may be admitted to hospital for traction.

D-i-y traction by gravity

Patients are sometimes advised to use gravity by hanging by the hands from a firmly fixed rail, a cross-beam or the top of a door frame, if they can do so safely and conveniently at home. Gripping the top of the door, or the door frame, they gradually raise their feet off the floor by bending their knees. This exercise applies traction to the shoulder joints as well as the spine. The duration of the exercise is limited by the patient's grip-endurance, or possibly by the endurance of the door.

Some traction appliances that work by gravity can be hired or bought to be used at home: the patient is strapped by the ankles to a horizontal frame which tilts backwards to some chosen angle, and the slope of the frame and the weight of the body produce the pull. Such a device should be used only on medical advice, as the pressure on the blood vessels in the head can harm someone with high blood pressure or a history of strokes or eye problems.

Movement

Exercise techniques are often important in the treatment of spinal conditions. They may be used as an adjunct to mobilising procedures, to enable the patient to maintain the restored range of movement and to strengthen muscles which have become weak through disuse or inhibition by pain.

Assisted or resisted exercises

Joints can become stiff if the muscles which move them are weak; by strengthening these, mobility can be increased. Since each joint movement involves the tensing of a set of muscles and the relaxation of the opposing set, assisted and resisted movement strengthens the muscle by working it in both directions of movement. Assisted movement is when you work your muscles but the therapist helps with the range and direction; resisted movement is when the therapist pushes against you doing the movement.

Proprioceptive neuromuscular facilitation (PNF)

PNF is a system of exercise which aims to obtain maximum muscle activity by using sensory and auditory stimuli to increase the response of the neuromuscular system. Resistance and stretch are also applied to groups of muscles.

In essence, the patient performs or tries to perform movements against the manual resistance offered by the therapist in certain spiral and diagonal patterns of movement. The movements contain elements of flexion (or extension) together with a rotatory component, and are closely related to normal functional movement. Maximum contraction of strong muscles is used to reinforce the effort of weaker muscles in the pattern. The specific placing of hands to apply pressure, the use of the voice to stimulate 'push' or 'pull', the stretching of muscles to initiate movement, are stimuli used to encourage movement. PNF procedures are normally done with the patient lying supine. It is hard work for therapist and patient.

Active exercises

These are of various kinds in which the patient takes over, following the therapist's instructions, in trying to mobilise joints and strengthen muscles.

The type of exercise prescribed depends on the patient's condition, on how long he has been out of action and on how fit he needs to be to return to normal life. What is suitable for one patient is not necessarily right for another.

If any exercise causes pain it may be aggravating the condition, so tell the physiotherapist when you find a movement painful. The exercise may have to be adjusted accordingly.

Some exercises are designed to strengthen and mobilise the spine when it is extended. Others strengthen the abdominal muscles; sideways bending and rotation (twisting) help to mobilise the spine. To do this, the therapist may provide manual or other resistance to particular movements. Spinal exercises are sometimes given in a hydrotherapy pool in warm water.

Some physiotherapy departments adopt the 'back school' approach in which exercises are carried out in groups. Classes with others help to raise morale and individuals can encourage and support each other. The competition often has a stimulating effect. Physiotherapists try to ensure that exercises match the age and needs of the individual.

If you have been taught to do the exercises and are expected to do them at home, make sure that you do them. Do them regularly and carefully, and for short periods at a time – if you have forgotten to do your morning session, do not do twice as much in the evening to catch up! Doing your exercises to music or while listening to a regular radio programme may help to remind and motivate you. If rest is suggested during or after a set of exercises, this is important and should not be skimped.

Isometric exercises

It is possible to contract the muscles very strongly but not move the joints at all; this happens in arm wrestling. This muscle action is called isometric exercise. The method has a particular benefit for back pain. Where inflammation of joints makes moving them painful, a special range of isometric exercises can be used which strengthen the muscles by bracing them without moving joints.

Electrotherapy

Physiotherapists are trained to administer several sorts of treatment which depend on the use of different types of electrical or electronic apparatus. Many people have found these therapies beneficial in relieving pain, though the effect is in some cases short-lived.

Ultrasound

This is used in treating injury to muscles, tendons and ligaments, but not bones. Ultrasonic therapy uses the energy of sound waves at very high frequencies, inaudible to human beings. The waves are applied to the affected area through a special apparatus. They penetrate the skin painlessly, and help to relax muscular spasm, and reduce swelling and relieve pain; they also promote healing in the tissues.

Short-wave and microwave diathermy

This is a method of relieving pain and stiffness in the deep tissues by applying high-frequency electromagnetic waves which cause heat in the tissues. Short-wave treatment affects deeper tissues than microwave. It is claimed to increase blood flow and to promote the body's repairing processes.

TENS (transcutaneous electrical nerve stimulation)

Severe chronic pain can sometimes be relieved by applying very small electrical currents to either side of the pain site. This method is thought to work by stimulating the nerve ends in the skin, and thus overriding the nervous system's reception of pain messages; its principles being the same as those of acupuncture.

Sufferers can administer this treatment by themselves, by means of a portable battery-operated unit, connected to electrodes which are attached to the skin with surgical tape. Such units cost from £80 upwards (some physio departments might loan them out). The wearer can switch the current on at any time, and control the amount, duration and strength of each dose of stimulation, which is felt as a gentle tingling. TENS is sometimes applied to a patient on complete bedrest. Some back pain sufferers swear by TENS, but it does not work for everybody. However, it is essential not to use a TENS machine unless you have first seen a physiotherapist or other health professional because its use may mask pain, the cause of which should be investigated.

Interferential therapy

This is another method of using electric current, via electrodes, attached to the skin around the painful area, to relieve pain by blocking the pain reception network, and to reduce inflammation by promoting better circulation. It may also be used to stimulate muscle contractions by applying a different frequency. The patient feels a tingling sensation, as in TENS.

Which kind of physiotherapy?

It is rare for a therapist to practise the full range of techniques. Some concentrate on gradual mobilisation, others on localised thrust manoeuvres, and yet others teach their patients to do active exercises. Each of these methods is beneficial to some patients, and found painful or troublesome by others.

Techniques and modalities of physiotherapeutic treatment are constantly being abandoned and resurrected and new ones appear regularly. Objective comparisons of different techniques are difficult: each one may work for some people but not for others.

CHAPTER 11

COMPLEMENTARY THERAPIES

MANY people seeking relief from back pain try out therapies which do not form part of orthodox medicine (although a number of doctors have had training in them, and practise them as a specialty).

You do not need to go through your GP to see an acupuncturist, osteopath, chiropractor, naturopath or shiatsu practitioner, but can consult one direct on your own responsibility. It may be wise to consult your GP beforehand, to ensure that there is no medical contra-indication in your case, though the therapist should tell you if your condition is not suitable for his treatment and ought to be seen by a doctor.

Practitioners in private practice can charge whatever fees they choose. It is wise, therefore, to ask beforehand what the charge is likely to be for your course of treatment.

Manipulative therapies

Some practitioners who are outside the system of state-registration carry out manipulative procedures similar to those of the orthodox repertoire. In some circumstances, manipulation is inadvisable or even dangerous, for example in the case of rheumatoid arthritis in the neck or an undiagnosed tumour.

Osteopathy and chiropractic are the main manipulative therapies used in treating the joints of the spine. In both, the first consultation may last an hour (and X-rays may be taken). The patient is thoroughly examined, asked to undertake a whole range of movements and the practitioner generally asks for details of the patient's medical – and life – history. Although manipulation forms the major treatment method of both osteopaths and chiropractors, these professions also make use of other approaches such as muscle re-education and the correction of postural faults.

Osteopathy

Osteopathy is a system of diagnosis and treatment for the mechanical problems which can affect all areas of the spine. Osteopaths use a variety of different manual techniques which are designed to improve the mobility and restore function to restricted spinal joints and the surrounding muscles and ligaments.

Treatment is generally painless and usually consists of soft tissue massage with gentle, passive stretching movements of the back. In some cases it is necessary to mobilise a very restricted joint using thrust techniques.

Osteopathic treatment is not available under the NHS, but a general practitioner may refer a patient to a medical practitioner with an osteopathic qualification or to an osteopath registered with the General Council and Register of Osteopaths (GCRO). There is no requirement for a doctor's referral: anyone can go to an osteopath direct. You can expect to pay between £15 and £25 for an initial session and between £10 and £20 for subsequent treatments. The cost may be higher in London.

In this country, training in osteopathic methods is provided by many institutions with varying lengths and content of courses. The British School of Osteopathy, the European School of Osteopathy and the British College of Naturopathy and Osteopathy run four-year full-time degree and diploma courses for people without medical qualifications wishing to train as osteopaths. Someone who has completed one of these courses can become a member of the GCRO, and the letters MRO after an osteopath's name and use of the title 'Registered Osteopath' indicate membership of the GCRO. The one-year course of the London College of Osteopathic Medicine is designed for qualified doctors who can then become members of the British Osteopathic Association and the GCRO.

It is advisable not to entrust yourself to any practitioner without checking his qualifications. Osteopathic techniques are practised in this country not only by trained osteopaths and by medical practitioners who have taken courses in osteopathy, but also by practitioners who are unqualified. The letters DO (diploma in osteopathy) on their own after someone's name may mean only a diploma obtained by post from a correspondence school, so it is important to look for the letters MRO (which denotes a registered osteopath) after the name of an osteopath who is not a doctor. The names of your local registered osteopaths can be obtained by telephoning the GCRO on (0734) 576585. Alternatively, the GCRO will send you a register of osteopaths if you write to them at 56 London Road, Reading, Berks RG1 4SQ (enclosing £2.50 and an s.a.e.).

Chiropractic
Chiropractors use a somewhat different range of manipulative techniques from osteopaths, although there are some features common to both. Osteopathy and chiropractic developed at about the same time in adjacent states in the U.S.A., and originally had different underlying theories: chiropractic emphasised the effect of misaligned joints on nerves, whereas osteopathy was concerned with treating joints to improve blood circulation. There were also some differences in approach: osteopaths tended to work more on muscles and tendons, and used leverage (e.g. twisting the body and putting pressure on shoulders and hips to adjust the lower back). Chiropractors tended to use direct pressure on the affected area. Today there is a lot of overlap between the two therapies, but chiropractors are more likely to use X-rays and other diagnostic tests.

There have been six formal government enquiries into chiropractic worldwide over the last 20 years. Each concluded that modern chiropractic therapy is safe when performed by an adequately trained chiropractor. Research published last year showed chiropractic in a favourable light. The study, funded by the British Medical Research Council, compared treatment of low back pain by chiropractors with hospital out-patient treatment (which included orthodox medical manipulation, stretching and exercise). The report concluded that chiropractic treatment gave better results which lasted longer, and was particularly effective for those with chronic or severe back pain.

The first visit to a chiropractor is usually spent diagnosing the problem, unless you're in intense pain and something can be done immediately. Usually, a course of between six and ten sessions is recommended. There are about 36 different adjustment techniques which chiropractors can use. Those most commonly used are short, rapid, shallow thrusts. One hand is placed directly over the joint to be adjusted, and a short sharp movement is made. It is a small, precise movement which should not be at all painful, although following initial treatment it is common to feel sore for a few days. A chiropractor may also use other techniques such as massage, ultrasound, or application of heat or cold to treat the muscles surrounding a joint.

A chiropractor who has taken a four-year full-time training course conforming to an internationally recognised standard of training, can become a member of the British Chiropractors' Association and be on its register. Send £2 and an s.a.e. (9 in × 6 in) for a copy of the register to the British Chiropractic Association, Premier House, 10 Greycoat Place, London SW1P 1SB. Treatment costs vary. On average, the initial session costs £18, subsequent ones £15. X-rays cost extra.

Naturopathy

Some naturopaths also practise manipulation and this may include osteopathic or chiropractic techniques. A naturopath treats ailments on the basis of the belief that healing depends on the correct action of the curative forces within the human organism. Illness is seen as a result of toxins accumulating in the system and symptoms of disease as the attempts of the body to throw off these harmful waste products. Naturopaths advocate correct diet and regulated activities as the means of maintaining good health, and discourage treatment by drugs.

After successfully completing the four-year full-time course from the British College of Naturopathy and Osteopathy, graduates are eligible to join the General Council and Register of Naturopaths and may be recognised by the letters ND, MRN. The General Council and Register of Naturopaths maintains a

register of practitioners who have satisfied their training requirements. Write to the Secretary of the GCRN, c/o Frazer House,
6 Netherhall Gardens, London NW3 5RR, enclosing £2 and a
large s.a.e. (27p). Alternatively, telephone 071-435 8728 to find
names of practitioners in your area.

Acupuncture

Acupuncture is an ancient Chinese therapy used in the treatment
of many diseases, as well as for the relief of pain. The principle of
acupuncture is the belief that in the human tissues there exist
numerous points connected with particular organs, and these
points are linked by a network of channels, called meridians,
through which streams of life energy flow. The functioning of an
organ is said to be affected by tapping these channels at appropriate points. In acupuncture, fine needles are inserted; other
ways of tapping the points include touch (acupressure), electric
currents, ultrasound and laser.

Western medicine rests on totally different assumptions, and
so finds it hard to account for the fact that acupuncture is
frequently effective. The probable explanation is that acupuncture leads the brain to produce substances called endorphins,
which act as a natural painkiller.

The initial diagnosis is very thorough. A considerable amount
of time will be spent asking the patient details about his general
condition. Questions may relate to physical, emotional and
energetic signs and symptoms. In addition, examination of the
tongue is a fundamental part of acupuncture diagnosis, as is the
taking of the 'pulses' – at both wrists and in three positions, by the
index, middle and ring fingers. The tongue and pulses give the
practitioner information about the condition of the body, and
indicate where the life energy needs to be changed.

In many places, acupuncture is available from private practitioners only, but some acupuncture is available at NHS pain relief
clinics. If you're seeing an acupuncturist privately, the cost of the
initial session will probably be between £20 and £35; subsequent
sessions will be between £15 and £22. Some general practitioners
are trained in and use acupuncture, and an increasing number of
chartered physiotherapists are using it. Members of the British
Medical Acupuncture Society are doctors trained in acupuncture;

the Society currently has nearly 700 members. For details, write to the Administrator, Newton House, Newton Lane, Lower Whitley, Warrington, Cheshire WA4 4JA (tel: 0925 73727). For physiotherapists, acupuncture is a postgraduate skill, and there is an Acupuncture Association of Chartered Physiotherapists. For details contact the Chartered Society of Physiotherapy (see page 76).

There is no one central regulatory body for acupuncture; there are a number of different organisations. The Council for Acupuncture holds a register of practitioners who are members of acupuncture associations approved by them. Also, the central office of the British Acupuncture Association keeps a list of qualified and registered acupuncturists and will provide a handbook and directory of members by writing (enclosing £2 and an s.a.e.) to BAAR, 34 Alderney Street, London SW1V 4EU (tel: 071-834 1012). Alternatively, the Institute for Complementary Medicine holds a national register of complementary practitioners who conform to their standards, and details can be obtained by writing to them (with an s.a.e.) at the Institute for Complementary Medicine, 21 Portland Place, London W1N 3AF. They can also provide addresses for the other therapies described in this section.

Shiatsu

This is a technique involving the application of pressure to acupuncture points and meridians. According to oriental medicine, deep pressure applied to certain points will have a similar effect to the use of needles, although the points may differ from the needle points. Shiatsu was originally the Japanese form of Chinese acupressure (see above), but has developed techniques of its own.

A shiatsu session can be expected to last between 45 minutes and an hour and a quarter. The first session usually begins with a history-taking and diagnosis, following a similar pattern to acupuncture. Treatment will be given by exerting pressure on several specific points, as well as general kneading massage. Pressure is applied in a great variety of ways. Sometimes the thumb or fingers are used, sometimes the palm or heel of the hand, or a knee or elbow. The intensity of pressure varies between gentle massage to a very strong pressure, but no more pain should be felt than that involved in the release of tension. Some shiatsu practitioners also use osteopathic and chiropractic techniques, based on energy movement.

Shiatsu can be used for the treatment of specific problems (including back pain), and also as a general preventive health measure. A register of practitioners who have fulfilled the minimum requirements of the Shiatsu Society can be obtained by writing (enclosing an s.a.e.) to the Shiatsu Society, 14 Oakdene Road, Redhill, Surrey RH1 6BT.

The cost of treatment will usually be somewhere between £15 and £25 for a session – the first one will probably be more expensive, and costs are highest in London.

CHAPTER 12

SURGERY

ON the whole, surgery is nowadays seldom suggested where some other treatment remains to be tried. Spinal surgery is usually the therapy of last resort, and should never be agreed to without serious consideration.

No surgeon can ever guarantee beforehand that a spinal operation will be a success, and complications, some serious, can sometimes occur. However, most operations are successful – otherwise surgeons would not continue doing them. The surgeon should discuss the position with you fully, and should give you some idea of what to expect after the operation. No operation is done without the patient's consent. A surgeon is unlikely to suggest an operation unless he is fairly sure of your full cooperation at all stages. To a large extent, success will call for your determination to regain strength and get back to normal.

Being successfully operated on does not mean that the spine is now as good as new, and that all previous activities can be resumed – including the ones that caused the original damage.

The spine is a complex structure, and it is seldom that damage such as a disc prolapse happens in isolation. It usually causes damage to other structures also, which will not be cured by the operation, and may go on causing problems afterwards. A complete recovery following a spinal operation is likeliest when the damage is the result of a single incident, and not the culmination of years of gradual deterioration.

If an operation is not a success, be wary of agreeing to a second one; statistics show that the chances of success grow less with each additional operation.

What an operation can do

There are three main reasons for operating: to relieve mechanical stress on the lumbar and sacral nerve roots; to stabilise one or more adjacent intervertebral joints when there is a mechanical weakness locally; and for intractable pain.

Where the surgeon cannot be certain whether he will have to remove a part of, or the whole of, a prolapsed disc or have to perform a spinal fusion, he may have to explore to find the cause of pain: this exploratory operation is called lumbar spondylotomy.

In rare cases, a disc prolapse is so massive as to be compressing the spinal cord, or damaging nerve roots; the effects, in addition to pain, can include weakness or loss of feeling in the legs, and partial or total incontinence. Then an operation to relieve the compression must be done with great urgency.

Discectomy

This operation is performed in order to free a nerve root. It is done under general anaesthesia. The removal of the prolapsed disc material may be all that is necessary, although the surgeon may decide to remove the whole of the disc nucleus, in order to prevent another prolapse.

He makes an incision in the ligamentum flavum, creating a window into the spinal canal (fenestration). He may remove a bit of the lamina, to improve surgical access.

Discectomy is not a serious operation, and often produces immediate relief from sciatic pain. The patient is usually allowed up almost at once and is encouraged to walk and bend; sometimes it is necessary to wear a corset for a few weeks. Most people are able to return to work, if it is sedentary, within a month or so; but if they do heavy work, they will not be able to return to it for at least two to three months.

In a few centres, orthopaedic surgeons and microsurgeons are speeding up recovery by doing the operation through a small cut and the use of a microscope. This is called microdiscectomy.

Sometimes the surgeon finds it necessary to remove bony thickening and osteophytes from the vertebral arch or body, if they are causing stretching, angulation, adhesion or compression of the nerve roots. The removal of bone from the articular processes of the vertebral arch is called facetectomy.

Spinal fusion

This operation is designed to stiffen a section of the spine, in order to prevent a deformity such as spondylolisthesis from increasing; to fix a section where movement is painful, such as a degenerated disc giving an abnormal pattern of movement, with secondary changes in the facet joints; or to stabilise the spine in an area weakened during surgery.

Most commonly, the operation consists of the laying down of a bone graft to increase the stability of the spine across one, two or three vertebrae. The bone for fusion is usually taken from the hip bone; this leaves no deformity or weakness.

Spinal fusion is a much more serious operation than disc-ectomy. Until a few years ago, it meant lying in a plaster shell for a month, and in bed for up to three months before being allowed up. Nowadays, however, this is less common. Some surgeons allow patients up after a week or two, provided there is nothing to contra-indicate this; a corset may have to be worn. Or if the bones are fixed together with wires, rods or screws, the patient may be allowed up after a day or two.

The back muscles may take quite a while to recover from the operation and to regain normal strength. The patient will later be given exercises by the physiotherapist to stabilise the spine and strengthen the muscles, and in a few months he could be back to full activity. But many patients take a year or more to recover completely. A lot depends on the patient: the physiotherapist will show the way but it is up to the patient to do the work.

Convalescence

There are some – but very few – convalescent homes to which patients can be sent after early discharge from hospital when they would have difficulty in going straight home to fend for themselves. The social worker at the hospital may be able to make the arrangements, with the consultant's support.

CHAPTER 13

OCCUPATIONAL THERAPY

PATIENTS may be referred to occupational therapy after recovering from surgery as part of rehabilitation, or after being inactive because of a prolonged spell of pain (where there was no surgery).

Patients are referred to occupational therapy in the same way as they are referred to physiotherapy. The two types of treatment are likely to overlap; the physiotherapist may start treating the patient when he is in bed, while occupational therapy does not start until he is up and out of bed.

Occupational therapy is a state registered profession supplementary to medicine. Occupational therapists who have completed their three or four year training are entitled to put Dip-COT after their name and also SROT if they choose to go on the state register. Occupational therapy is usually requested in the first instance by the consultant or other doctor, but the actual treatment is left to the discretion of the therapist. It may take the form of any activity, work or recreation which will most effectively help the patient to achieve full recovery and return to work; or which will minimise the effects of permanent disability and help him to live with such a disability.

How OT helps

Occupational therapy for patients with back problems is mainly re-educative. The occupational therapist will be concerned to help the patient learn to manage his own body, to realise the limitations imposed by his condition, to avoid actions which bring on back pain, and to learn new ways of carrying out everyday activities, so as not to aggravate his back. This can include teaching him how to bend, how to lift, and giving advice on more suitable seating and better work positions.

In nearly all occupational therapy departments, there is an area with a kitchen, a bathroom and a bedroom, where patients are not only taught safer ways of carrying out activities, but will also practise them under supervision, until these techniques become automatic. It is not easy to change the patterns of movement of a lifetime without professional help.

If the house you live in is badly designed for a person with back trouble, the occupational therapist from the hospital, or one from the local authority social services department, may visit and recommend adaptations. The social services department may be able to provide financial help to carry them out.

Rehabilitation and returning to work

In the case of a patient who is still attending hospital when he is almost fit for work, the occupational therapist may help by analysing his job requirements, and suggesting ways of lessening back strain.

If you ought to be doing light work for a time, the doctor can write to your firm's personnel manager or medical officer, setting out what is needed. Do not hesitate to ask the doctor to do this.

When, because of your back, there is no hope of your returning to your original work and your employers are unable to offer an alternative lighter job, you can ask the disablement resettlement officer (DRO) at the local jobcentre for advice and help which might include retraining for a more suitable job.

CHAPTER 14

PREVENTING A RECURRENCE

FOR people who have already experienced one episode of back trouble, the probability of being struck by an acute attack of back pain is higher than for people who have never yet been troubled. This is because an attack, regardless of what caused it, tends to leave the victim with a degree of damage to the tissues, or with a weaker back and abdominal muscles than before.

Back schools
There are a growing number of back schools, usually attached to physiotherapy departments in hospitals. They offer a form of educational therapy first developed in Sweden for back pain sufferers. It consists of instruction on how to use the body, actively and posturally. Anatomy of the spine and descriptions of the causes of back pain are included. Advice on the layout, planning and design of work – ergonomics – is also given. The lesson is simple: the better you understand your back, the more readily you can cope when it is painful.

Advice on posture
Many of us acquire minor postural deformities which lead to avoidable backache and which can be treated: for example, the tendency to a rounded back, head poked forward and shoulders tensed up. If this is due to muscular weakness and stiffness, exercises should help. But often it is just a matter of habit. Old habits should therefore be shed and new ones learned, and postural advice on a new way of using your body can help.

The Alexander Technique

The Alexander Technique is a method of postural re-education. Fundamental to the technique, which is nearly 100 years old, is the concept of 'use' of the body. Rather than focusing on specific problems (e.g. back pain), the overall use of the body is looked at, and the aim is to increase the pupil's awareness of balance, posture and movement in everyday activity. For example, habitual slouching when sitting would be seen as harmful body use. It is believed that for each of us there is an optimum posture and way of moving. This unfortunately becomes overlaid with bad habits which then feel natural to us. The task of the Alexander teacher is to make the pupil more aware of his physical self, to enable him to positively direct his body towards using it in a better way.

In practice, the Alexander Technique is taught by a teacher making small physical adjustments to the pupil's body and some accompany these with particular verbal directions. These lessons enable the pupil to acquire a sense of what the correct position feels like (often this will feel 'wrong' because it goes against habit).

The Alexander Technique is taught on a one-to-one basis, as people have individual habits. It is possible to find group classes which give a general idea of how the technique works; some adult education institutes have such courses available. Individual sessions can cost between £8 and £18 for half an hour, the cost being higher in London, and teachers recommend a course of about ten lessons initially, taken fairly closely together.

There are specialist teachers who have undergone a three-year training course under the auspices of the Society of Teachers of the Alexander Technique (STAT). Before going to an Alexander teacher you may want to check that he or she is a member of STAT or one of its affiliated bodies, such as NASTAT (North American Society of Teachers of the Alexander Technique) or AUSTAT (Australian Society of Teachers of the Alexander Technique). You can write to STAT for a list of teachers (enclosing an s.a.e.) at 10 London House, 266 Fulham Road, London SW10 9EL (tel: 071-351 0828).

Feldenkrais Method

The Feldenkrais Method is concerned with creating a greater awareness of patterns of movement, the aim being a gradual re-education leading to greater freedom of movement and enhanced comfort. The method has its roots in Western science (physics and mechanical engineering) and Eastern martial arts (judo), as its founder, Dr Moshe Feldenkrais was highly trained in both. The focus is on learning to recognise ways of moving or holding the body which are restrictive and habitual and on discovering new options which are more efficient and graceful. The re-learning process is facilitated by the use of gentle movements, done at a pace and intensity that does not involve force or pain. The lessons usually begin lying or sitting on the floor and involve new perceptions of walking, crawling, the natural movements of babies, awareness of breathing while moving and the way in which the head, eyes, spine and limbs move in relation to one another.

The method is taught in two different formats: as a series of lessons, called Awareness through Movement, through which a teacher leads a group in classes or workshops; and as one-to-one lessons called Functional Integration. If you are suffering from a back problem, the classes may be helpful as the movements are done very gently. It is important to inform the teacher of your problem beforehand; some even offer special classes for those with back pain. If your back trouble is acute, it may be advisable to have individual lessons. These cost from £15–£30 for a one hour lesson. Any specific difficulties will be explored in the context of the functioning of the entire nervous system, taking into account the fact that a back problem can be related to a pattern of use in other parts of the body, the eyes, or the feet, for example.

To obtain a directory of teachers of the Feldenkrais Method, write (enclosing an s.a.e.) to the Feldenkrais Guild, PO Box 370, London N10 3XA. In September 1990, 24 new teachers graduated from the first UK-based training programme.

Signs and warnings

Having once been afflicted, you should be able to recognise some of the danger signs; perhaps a stab of pain in a muscle, or a tingling in the fingers or toes, warning you that you must stop something you are doing, or change some posture you are maintaining. If you know of something in your daily routine that triggered off the original trouble, and you have not changed your ways, do so now. This may involve changing your leisure activities, or even your job – temporarily, or even permanently. Even if this possibility raises great difficulties, it needs to be considered seriously. Traditionally, it is thought that people who refuse to 'give in' to back pain are the very ones who are most likely to be plagued by repeated attacks. This could result in the underlying condition, which caused the attacks, becoming chronic. (In medical language, chronic means long-term.)

A recent approach by some doctors to patients' attitude to pain is to advise tackling it more directly. Many people live in fear of pain. This is perfectly normal and understandable but, pain being a common experience, exaggerated fears may need investigation and unravelling. Often the medical profession itself has tended to encourage people's fear of pain, advising rest when, perhaps, encouragement to get going might have been wiser.

The chronic sufferer

When certain changes have occurred in the structure of the spine, especially if these are the outcome of a degenerative process, there is no way of restoring all the functions of a normal spine.

Sometimes people have to be told that there is nothing more that can be done in the way of medical treatment for their back trouble, and find that treatment by physiotherapists or other therapists does not ease their suffering. They must then learn to live with their faulty spine, since they cannot be given a new one.

Such advice is bound to be depressing, even when accompanied by the assurance that there is no serious organic disease.

Moreover, chronic pain can itself be depressing. Some people in this situation let the rest of their life be dominated by their back; others are more able to meet the challenge and learn to cope.

Trying anything
Although a patient may have been told that all the normal measures have been tried, there is always a possibility that the

verdict may become outdated by new knowledge, improved diagnostic techniques and methods of treatment not previously available.

Some sufferers, therefore, feel that there is always a chance that another surgeon, another doctor, another therapist, may have a way of doing something for them. There are a number of doctors and other therapists in private practice who offer specialist treatment of back pain. They are generally exponents of a particular line of therapy and if that does not work are therefore unlikely to propose alternatives. The main advantage in seeing someone privately is that you may be seen more quickly and may be buying more time with the particular practitioner.

Other long-term sufferers pin their faith on a succession of non-orthodox treatments which may be providing no more than brief temporary relief. There is probably no harm in this as long as they are seeing a professionally qualified person, even though it is unlikely that one of these treatments will provide a cure, or restore to their spine all its former mobility.

The constant trying out of this treatment or that remedy is likely to set up an endless cycle of hope and disappointment. Miracle cures are mainly anecdotal. There is, moreover, some risk that, for instance, regular manipulation may accelerate osteoarthritis of facet joints.

Making the best of things

A chronic back sufferer can do much to help himself. First of all, there are almost certainly alternative ways of tackling any particular job which cause less spinal stress and are therefore less painful, and which are physically more efficient. Also, it is possible to alter or redesign your working environment with the aim of minimising postural stress on the spine: by adjusting the height of a working surface, by changing your own posture, by choosing a different chair or desk.

There are a number of aids to back comfort, some designed for the disabled, which can be used to make life more independent. The Disabled Living Foundation (380 Harrow Road, London W9 2HU, telephone 071-289 6111), can provide information on what special equipment is available and where it can be obtained.

The National Back Pain Association (write, enclosing s.a.e. to 31-33 Park Road, Teddington, Middlesex TW11 0AB, telephone 081-977 5474) is a registered charity whose aim is to promote research into the causes, treatments and prevention of back pain, and to increase understanding of how the problem of back pain can be avoided. The membership fee of £10 a year includes subscription to a quarterly newsletter, *Talkback*, with information about the Association's activities and research projects, and other relevant publications. Local groups of back pain sufferers have been set up in some places under the NBPA's auspices.

Pain clinics

If you have chronic back pain which you are finding hard to cope with, your GP may refer you to a pain clinic run under the auspices of the NHS. A number of services are offered at such a clinic, although the particular range varies from health authority to health authority. Advice on painkilling drugs will be given, suitable physiotherapy techniques, occupational therapy, and counselling may also be available. Some clinics employ acupuncturists who specialise in pain relief, and TENS machines (see p. 82) may be used.

Self Help in Pain (SHIP, Whitstable) is a self-help group offering group support, advice and counselling to people suffering from chronic pain. For details send an s.a.e. to SHIP, 33 Kingsdown Park, Tankerton, Kent CT5 2DT.

What you can do to help yourself

It is important to identify positively the things that do not make matters worse, and to concentrate on them as a basis for an improvement of life. Assuming you can find some activity – such as short walks or swimming, or simple exercises which do not upset your back – do it regularly, a bit more and a bit faster or farther every day. Almost any exercise (not jogging!) will do to start with, as the basis for improvement, and help you to become generally more physically fit.

People who are physically fit are generally able to tolerate pain better than the unfit. Their sensation of pain may be no different but if affects them less and they are better able to ignore it.

Some of the things you can do which should make your life easier include:

- keep a check on your weight; extra pounds mean extra stress on the spine
- eat a healthy balanced diet
- learn to relax
- learn to live according to a routine, and plan ahead, so that you never need to rush
- give careful consideration to the movements or actions which aggravate your symptoms and try to avoid them
- when you have a 'good' day, do not try to catch up on all the neglected things: having further weeks of misery because you rushed to do too much on the 'good' day is not worth it
- make sure that you have a suitable chair and bed – ask advice from the physiotherapist, occupational therapist or osteopath before buying new furniture
- keep active. Rest is appropriate for acute back pain; chronic back pain tends to benefit from the right kind of exercise, preferably of the most enjoyable type and as strenuous as you can manage
- change patterns and positions as needed to ensure that your sex life can continue on as regular a basis as possible. Prolonged back pain can have a devastating effect on sexual activity. Back pain can also be used (often unconsciously) as an excuse for not engaging in sexual activity. The situation deserves understanding and sympathetic analysis from both partners. Postures can be experimented with. For example, experimenting which partner is on top; side to side positions; one partner sitting on a chair, the other astride.

The future for back trouble

Back trouble – chiefly in the form of low back pain – has taken on some of the aspects of an epidemic in the western world; that is to say, though it is not an infectious complaint, its incidence is seen to be constantly increasing. In Britain, it creates a demand for treatment which represents an ever-increasing burden on the health services. Analysis of current trends suggests that in the next 25 years this burden is likely to double. The already huge number of working days lost each year would also be likely to increase in proportion. The sum of all the individual misery that back trouble causes may, shortly, represent a luxury that this country cannot afford.

It would seem, therefore, that back pain sufferers of the future are more likely to be offered short shrift and grudging sympathy by doctors and employers alike. Harsh though this may seem, it has some backing from some advanced medical opinion.

Pain avoidance and pain confrontation

The latest approaches to the problem of back pain take their stand on the fact that most back pain is self-limiting; in 80 to 90 per cent of cases, an attack will clear up within six weeks at most, whether it is left alone or treated, and regardless of the form that any treatment takes.

Nor, it is claimed, does it make much difference whether the patient adopts the conventional method of bed rest (referred to as 'pain avoidance') or simply carries on with his usual activities as best he can (called 'pain confrontation'). Recovery is said to be, if anything, more likely to be rapid with the latter approach.

The disability factor

Back pain, in this view, is not really on the increase. What is increasing to epidemic proportions is people's readiness to expect medical treatment for it and an increased incidence of 'back pain disability' – an illness in which psychological factors play as important a part as physical ones. It manifests itself in acceptance of invalidity, which means staying away from work, retiring to bed, requesting sickness certificates and extensive treatment. It is a self-reinforcing condition, in that the more the sufferer gives way to it and comes to see himself as an invalid, the worse are his chances of recovery.

This is even more the case if he undergoes a variety of treatments, including surgery, which fail to bring about satisfactory relief; each successive treatment carries a reduced chance of success, and leads to a further retreat into invalidism.

It is pointed out that with improvements in medical care in less advanced parts of the world, back pain disability increases, because people who would previously have had to put up with their discomfort till it went away, are encouraged to seek medical help, seeking immediate relief or cure.

Attitudes to pain

At the root of this search for medical help is said to be the psychological problem of the fear of pain. Attitudes to pain are highly subjective, and conditioned by each person's individual psychology, which is the product of many different factors. Thus tolerance of pain varies enormously, and the identical kind of pain provokes widely different reactions.

The confrontationalists believe that an acute condition is most likely to become chronic in people who are least able or willing to tolerate pain, because prolonged rest and the avoidance of most exertion are not curative, but debilitating. Muscles, joints and bones deteriorate so that each exertion becomes progressively harder, in a sort of vicious circle; and a weakened physique also predisposes to further injury. Psychologically, too, the motivation towards effort and exertion becomes progressively fainter.

So the treatment of back pain in the future seems likely to take the form of encouraging the patient to refuse to give way to his pain and, by so doing, to limit its duration and effect.

A similarly vigorous approach to back pain is seen in a new exercise method being developed in Denmark. It is designed to strengthen the back and shoulder muscles, which are said to grow weak because modern living causes them to be underused. Contrary to accepted notions, patients are advised to start the exercises while still suffering an acute attack of pain; but the exercises are claimed to be equally beneficial in cases of chronic pain. They are also said to have preventive value.

This new method received a lot of publicity a couple of years ago, and there was controversy over how safe it was as it had not undergone controlled trials. In general, if you are suffering from back pain you should not attempt vigorous exercise unless you are being seen by a chartered physiotherapist or other health professional, who can advise you as to the suitability for you of particular exercises, and can monitor their effect.

CHAPTER 15

TAKING CARE OF YOUR BACK

FEW people give a thought to their spine until they are suffering the consequences of not thinking. When you find yourself squatting to reach a low cupboard because you cannot bend your aching back, you become aware that you should have learned to squat in the first place.

Everyone should learn the basic rules of looking after the spine. If you have never felt so much as a twinge, following these rules should help to ensure that you never will. If you have already suffered a bout of back trouble, they should help to prevent recurrences.

If this trouble has left you with some permanent problem, you will hardly need telling to treat your back with respect. But if you now feel perfectly all right, 'as good as new', avoid the false optimism of thinking you can now resume all your old ways. Once you have had back trouble, you are rather more likely to have it again, unless you take deliberate measures to prevent this.

This is not to say that you should become excessively anxious about yourself, or avoid every sort of activity. On the contrary, it is important that you should be as active as possible.

Without physical activity, the body becomes weak and unstable, and without movement it becomes stiff. The mobility of the spine and the resilience of its joints and ligaments are essential functions. Without them, the spine would be more readily strained and would lose its shock-absorbing capacity. Even more important are the muscles: not only those of the back but all those which support the spine, including the abdominal muscles.

Without muscular support, the spine is unstable and easily injured.

Every one of your daily activities needs to be reviewed in the light of what you know about the structures of your back, and how they are affected by bending, twisting, and even keeping still.

Lying in bed

If you never need to give your back a thought when you wake up in the morning; if there is no stiffness or pain when you roll over, sit up, and get out of bed, then your bed is probably all right for you – no matter how it looks to other people.

But if you wake up with a feeling of stiffness which does not disperse until you have been moving around for a while, the cause may simply be your bed.

Mattress

A very soft or sagging mattress makes your vertebral column sag, stretching the ligaments that support it. This matters less if you change position frequently in your sleep, but if you tend to lie all night in one position, these ligaments may be strained. A soft mattress which allows you to sink deeply into it may even discourage you from moving about.

Even people whose back does not normally trouble them, find that a soft bed leaves them feeling stiff in the morning. A good bed should support the body evenly, and be easy to move about on.

If you decide to buy a new bed, choose one with a firm or solid base; avoid a base which is soft or springy. Choose a reasonably firm mattress: it is better to buy one which feels a little too hard, rather than one which is too soft. So-called 'orthopaedic' mattresses tend to be more expensive than ordinary firm mattresses, without having any special advantages.

If the bed you have is too soft, you can make it firmer by putting a board under the mattress, provided that the mattress itself is not disintegrating with age. The board should be as wide as the bed base and at least as long as the distance from your head to your buttocks.

Pillows

Arrange the pillows in the way that seems to you most comfortable. A pillow placed between the head and shoulders needs to support the neck rather than the head. There is seldom any need to buy special pillows.

But too many pillows, or too thick a pillow, would push the head up, stretching the neck; and while you are asleep, the neck is then apt to bend sideways or forwards and the spine to become flexed. The neck vertebrae should always be kept in a continued line with the vertebrae of the chest.

Lying on your back with the head resting on a 'butterfly' pillow supports the head and stops it lolling from side to side. Simply tying a folded towel round your neck may also do the trick. (You can make a butterfly pillow by taking a thin or loosely-filled pillow and shaking the filling down each end, then twisting the pillow in the centre or tying it in half.) You may find it necessary to place another pillow underneath.

For someone who needs lots of pillows at night because of a bad chest, it is best to organise the support so that the whole spine rests on an incline. You may be able to do it with pillows; or it may be possible to incline the whole bed by raising the legs at the head on to blocks. The aim is to keep the whole spine, trunk and head in line with each other.

Getting dressed

Someone who is already suffering from back trouble may find it best to wear clothes which can be put on and taken off without much bending or arm raising. Gadgets are available to help spinal sufferers with putting on difficult garments such as tights, socks and shoes. When bending down to tie shoe laces causes a problem, this can be solved by sitting on a chair with a supportive back, and bending the hip and knee to bring the foot up to within reach – that is, using hip and knee movement instead of back movement.

Standing

For a correct stance, lift the top of your head keeping your chin tucked in. As well as standing tall, you should stand relaxed. Standing still for a long period can be uncomfortable for someone not used to it, and it is then easy to sag, so increasing the fatiguing effect by straining the muscles. However, except for soldiers on parade, standing still is rarely necessary. Mostly, we are free to look about, move our hands and shift from one foot to another, and so any given stance is seldom maintained for long. Consciously pulling in your abdomen is helpful.

One remedy for postural stress is to change position. If you cannot, and the job calls for work with one hand only, use the other hand to lean on. When you use both hands and are standing at a work bench, table or sink, ideally you should be able to rest your pelvis or stomach against it, with one foot forward in line with your hands, so that you have a balanced posture.

Washing hair and shaving

Leaning forward over a dressing-table or washbasin to see in a mirror may become a cause of backache. It can be avoided by bringing the mirror nearer, either putting it on an extension arm or fixing it on the wall beside the basin. While shaving, the fact that your arms are raised increases the workload on the back if you have to bend forward. For arranging your hair, the mirror need not be so close, but must be at a suitable height. If you have to stoop to see in the mirror, raise it farther up the wall.

Bending over a basin to wash your hair puts undue stress on both the neck and the back. It may help to sit on a stool and rest your elbows on the side of the basin or sink. A better way is to wash the hair under the shower. If necessary, you can buy an inexpensive shower attachment to fit on to the bath taps, and wash your hair while bathing.

Just sitting

When sitting at leisure, the important thing is to get the buttocks well back into the chair because sitting slouched in a chair may flex the lumbar region more than any other movement or posture. Some back sufferers are more comfortable if they avoid crossing their knees and sit with their feet and knees well apart.

If the chair is soft and does not give enough support, put a cushion at the small of the back. Some people with back trouble prefer high-backed chairs, but lumbar support is more important than support at shoulder level.

Choose a chair that is the right height for you: your feet should be planted on the floor, not dangling in space. Avoid a very low chair as this can put undue strain on your back when you get up out of the chair.

A pamphlet *Are you sitting comfortably?* available (free, but send an s.a.e.) from the Arthritis and Rheumatism Council, 41 Eagle Street, London WC1 4AR, telephone 071–405 8572 describes what to look for when choosing an easy chair.

Back shops

There are specialist shops throughout the country which supply goods (e.g. furniture, pillows) specifically for people with back problems. When possible, try something out in the shop before buying it; otherwise, see if you can buy it on approval, so you can return it if you find it is not suitable for you. The National Back Pain Association (for address see p. 101) produces an information sheet which lists back shops throughout the country.

Sitting when working

The seat of the chair for working should be deep enough (front to back) so that the thighs are supported, and the front edge of the seat should not dig into the thigh; this could cause pressure on the sciatic nerve. The chair seat should be inclined about 5 degrees to the horizontal, forwards, and be high enough for the knee angle to be not less than 90 degrees when the feet are flat on the ground.

The back rest of a typist-chair should be adjustable so that the height above the seat can be varied to provide support at the lumbar part of the spine. Where there is a full-length back rest, it should be contoured to give support at the lumbar level.

Office work often requires both writing and typing, and each requires a different posture. Since the height of office desks can seldom be varied, it should be possible to raise and lower the chair.

Typing imposes a fair amount of strain on the back, particularly the neck and upper back, and also on the shoulders, because the typist often has to sit for longish periods with the arms unsupported. Therefore, for typing you should sit higher than for writing; the typewriter should be at a height that allows the

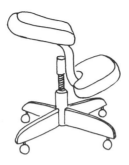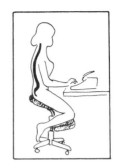

upper arms to hang relaxed, with only the weight of the forearms having to be lifted. You should sit as close to the typewriter as you can without cramping your movements. If you sit too far from it, you have to lift the whole arm forward to reach it, increasing the strain on the upper back.

A new style of chair is now widely available, which looks rather like a prie-dieu, but the upper cushion is for sitting on; it is tilted foward, and your knees rest on the lower cushion. There is no back support, but because some of your weight is taken by your knees and thighs, your back naturally assumes the correct lumbar curve. Chairs of this sort may be found specially comfortable when no back support is required; for example, for typing – but not all day long. Several versions are available, some with adjustable height.

Desks and other equipment

Chairs used for work are only satisfactory if the working environment in which they are used is also well designed. Even if your working chair allows you to sit supported in the right places, with the spine in a balanced neutral position and freedom to make regular minor changes in posture, the work itself may make it less than satisfactory, if ergonomics have not been taken into account.

For a given situation, at work or at leisure, the key factors are

● the angle of vision, and the need for subsidiary movements of the head

- the position of the hands relative to the seat and feet and
- the support of the body.

When work is laid out on a flat surface, the angle of vision is downwards and it is necessary to bend the head. To avoid this, designers, architects, artists and draughtsmen work on tilted surfaces.

For other people, to avoid bending the head forward when reading, the book or paper needs to be propped up. Rather than sitting with head bent when paperwork such as ledgers, computer print-outs or working drawings have to be flat on the desk, it is better to lean forward supporting oneself on the table or desk with the elbows.

For writing, the desk should be high enough to allow the knees to tuck right under it, and let you sit fairly upright. But not so high as to strain the arms and shoulders; that is, not much above elbow height when sitting relaxed.

If a lot of reading or writing has to be done, a tilted desk is best. Where such a desk is not available, a drawing board propped up slantwise on books can provide a substitute. It is also possible to buy a special sloped writing surface.

Typists and VDU operators risk postural stress by repeatedly bending the neck down and sideways to look at whatever they are copying. This can be avoided if the material to be copied is raised and placed centrally – for instance, on an inclined clipboard, reading stand or lectern, behind the keyboard.

Try not to sit still for long periods; get up and walk about now and again.

Housework

With any task, in and out of the house, it is the length of time spent in any one position, as well as the effort imposed on the back, that counts. It is a good idea to change tasks (and therefore positions) fairly often. Any activity where repetitive bending is required may cause trouble, particularly if it becomes fatiguing. Instead of doing one job until the bitter end, it may be possible to alternate it with another. For example, instead of spending a whole afternoon standing up ironing, leave half of it until later on, and do something else meanwhile.

If you have had back trouble, learn to delegate some or all of the heavier jobs that were formerly your lot. Make all able-bodied members of the family pull their weight.

Bed making is a job that often makes a painful back worse, and in some cases even induces back trouble, because it requires a good deal of bending and stretching. Ideally, the bed should be high enough for the mattress to be at hip height, narrow enough for you to reach across easily, and placed so that you can walk all round.

On the old-fashioned high bedstead, it requires less effort to make the bed than on a low divan bed. A low bed can be raised by putting blocks or bricks under the legs.

When making the bed, get close to it and bend at the hips and knees, keeping your back upright. If you have any difficulty in bending at hips and knees, kneel down when tucking in the bedclothes.

A fitted bottom sheet and a duvet do away with the need to bend to tuck in bedclothes. When changing a fitted sheet, do not stretch over the bed, but kneel close to each corner of the bed in turn.

A mattress should be turned by someone else. If you really have to do it yourself, have handles fitted to the sides (at the ends, too, if it is to be turned fore and aft). Grasp the handles and lift the side of the mattress so that you stand erect; back away a step and then step up on to the base and raise the mattress high enough to turn it over by letting it fall over to the other side. But better to leave it to other members of the household to do the turning.

Cleaning the bath puts considerable strain on the back. This job can be done much more easily by kneeling beside the bath and leaning across to rest one hand on the far edge of the bath to take your body weight, or by sitting on a chair alongside. A long-handled sponge or mop is useful. A bath is cleaned more easily when still warm immediately after use, so keep cleaning materials at hand – and insist that the others in the household clean the bath themselves.

You can avoid cleaning the bath altogether. Various preparations are available (especially for bathing children) which replace soap, and leave no ring round the bath. Or, if you prefer to wash with soap, putting a squirt of washing-up liquid in the bath water will ensure that there will be no ring.

Cleaning the floor and using a vacuum cleaner can be stressful to the back, so do it in short sessions. Make sure that the handle is long enough for you. Some cylinder cleaners have extension pieces; fitting one of these may help. When vacuuming, use your legs and your body weight to do the work. Always pull forwards and backwards in short lengths. Avoid twisting movements. Above all, do not just stand and make your arms do the work: that way is bound to stress your back.

Similarly, when using a mop, carpet sweeper or broom, move the whole body forwards and backwards with the sweeping action, not just bending from the waist to get the increased reach.

Dusting gives you opportunities for different kinds of muscle action. It is a good idea to slot short spells of it into spells of vacuuming, polishing, washing floors or any other task which requires vigorous movement in one direction only, for which you generally use your stronger arm. Try using the other arm or use both arms and stretch upwards to counteract the bending and pushing movements of vacuuming.

In the kitchen, have at hand all the things you use regularly – for instance, saucepans on the wall, plates and dishes at waist height. Only the things you use least often, or which are fairly light, should be stowed away below thigh height in low cupboards or out of easy reach above chest height. Ideally, heavy equipment such as a food mixer or cast iron casserole should be kept where it need not be lifted to be got out.

Whenever you have to do anything near floor level, get right down to it. Bend your knees to lift dishes in and out of the oven or dishwasher. When lifting a heavy casserole, hold it close to your body, with your elbows bent. To save your back, do it in stages: put a stool at the side of the oven, squat down, put the casserole on the stool, stand up and lift the casserole on to the top of the cooker or working surface.

Having a tall stool in the kitchen is a good idea so that you can alternate between sitting and standing. A stool should have a foot-rail and needs to be of a height to suit the height of the work surface.

Work surfaces

The height of work surfaces – sink, draining board, table or working area – matters a great deal. The correct height varies with the job being done, as well as from person to person. The surface should be high enough so that you do not have to bend forwards, but not so high that you have to hunch your shoulders in order to do the job. A cooker or a kitchen unit can be raised by being put on a plinth.

If you are too tall for washing up without stooping over the sink, raise the washing-up bowl by putting it on a small wooden stand, or on top of another upturned bowl, or on the draining board. If the surface is too high for you, try standing on a small step (made out of an inverted box, perhaps) while working there, but you could hurt yourself by forgetting about the box and stepping off unwittingly.

Ideally, it would be better to rearrange your kitchen so that the worktops are the correct height. The top of a sink should be at about elbow height, but work surfaces and the top of a cooker should be two or three inches lower. It is important to stand close to the work surface.

Less standing

You may be able to cut down on cooking: by the use of a microwave oven and a freezer, you can abolish lengthy standing at a conventional hob, do away with heavy metal saucepans, reduce washing up. Having a reserve of frozen dishes means that there can be a hot meal even when your back is playing you up: but be sure to have an upright freezer, not the cavernous chest type.

Many domestic activities (preparing food, washing up, ironing) can be be done seated. There is no law that says you have to stand to iron. Alter the height of the board to relate to your sitting position. It is important not to have it too high because having the arms continually raised imposes strain on the shoulders, neck and upper back.

Washing clothes

When washing by hand, do not use a sink or basin that makes you stoop: it is better to put a bowl at the right height for you in the sink or on the draining board.

Wet clothes and bed linen are much heavier than dry ones: lifting wet sheets and towels in and out of a low washing machine is the sort of movement that might eventually cause back trouble. When taking clothes out of a front-loading washing machine, put a low chair or stool beside the machine. Put a basket or large bowl on the floor, and squatting down, pull the washing into it. Then carefully lift the basket on to the stool. Do this in stages; try to make sure that you lift only one piece of wet washing at a time. If transferring something heavy such as a large wet bathtowel to the spin drier of a twin–tub machine, do it one end at a time.

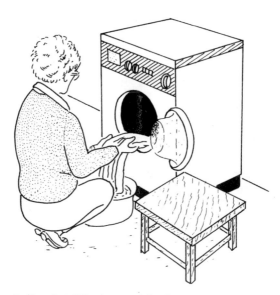

Squat with a straight back to reach low items; e.g. to load or unload a washing machine

Looking after babies and young children

A cot with a drop-side makes it easier to lift a child in and out; choose a cot high enough to save you having to stoop. Bringing the child's weight as close to the adult's body as possible reduces the amount of effort required.

When lifting a toddler from the ground, bend your knees and go down to him and lift him close to you. Swinging a child up at arms' length can be a cause of acute back trouble.

With a rucksack type of baby carrier where the child is placed behind the parent, its weight is taken through the shoulders and across the back of the hips. If possible, get someone to lift the carrier on for you, or find a safe place to prop it and the baby, while you get it on to your shoulders.

When bathing a small baby in a baby bath, put the bath on a table where you can stand or sit without stooping. Do not try to empty the bath yourself if you have a vulnerable back, because water is heavy to carry, and baby baths are an awkward shape to lift. Get some able-bodied person to do it for you. If none is available, bale out the water gradually with a jug. This will mean several trips and is laborious, but better than injuring your back.

When dressing a child, put him on a chair or bed to avoid undue bending. For doing up shoe laces, the foot should be put up on to a box or chair. Do not stoop – squat or kneel.

Lifting, shifting and carrying

Injuries can be caused by the unexpected: the box which was full when you thought it was empty, mistiming when lifting something jointly with another person, the load which you did not know was stuck.

The secret of safe lifting is to avoid static heaving and to use your body weight.

Stand properly: when you lift or shift an object, get as close to it as possible, with feet around it rather than to one side or behind it. Stand so that you are firmly balanced, one foot ahead of the other, ready to move off in the right direction.

To get a good grip on the load, bend the hips and knees until it can be reached, then grasp it firmly. If there is nothing on the load by which to hold it, use a sling, or ropes.

Technique of lifting

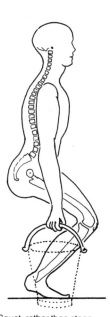

Let the leg muscles do the work

1. Squat, rather than stoop, to grasp the load

2. Straighten the back so that it is in the line of gravity, then let the leg muscles do the lifting

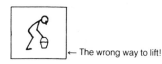

← The wrong way to lift!

Lifting, heaving or carrying with arms outstretched throws needless strain on the chest, upper back and shoulders – so keep the load close to your body. A weight held out at arms' length causes as much stress on the spine as ten times that weight held close to the side, hence the risk when lifting a box out of a car boot. The shorter the lever, the smaller the effort required, so the closer one can get to the object, the better.

When dealing with something large and heavy, lift it first at one end only, and get it on to a higher level before you take the full load. This halves the stress.

When putting things down, if you cannot safely drop the object (which is the best way), put the lifting drill into reverse. Keep the object close to your body, watch your fingers and put one end or corner down first.

Rather than carrying a heavy load, pull it on a trolley or, if that is not possible, divide it into two smaller loads – one for each hand – or make a second journey.

Whatever you are lifting or carrying, keep its centre of gravity as near as you can over or under your own centre of gravity. This means that you have to keep your knees apart enough to keep the load close to you, and must use your leg muscles to help lift. Before you actually lift, it is a good idea to check quickly that your back is in the correct posture, then look up and tuck your chin in. (Do not tackle a lifting job with your back rotated, twisted or bent sideways.)

Using your body weight can help to move things and saves the stress of direct muscular effort. If you move the body to give it momentum, it has what is called kinetic energy, and you can transfer that energy to something else. Just as you can give a cricket ball movement and thus kinetic energy enough to break a window, you can use your body in such a way that energy is transferred to the load you wish to shift. In this way, stress on the spine is reduced.

Do not ever attempt to shift a heavy cupboard or chest by yourself. If furniture has to be moved, try to get help. Unload every single item from the cupboard on to a convenient table before moving the cupboard – laborious but safer.

When pushing or pulling, make use of your legs and body weight. If the object to be moved is high and stable enough, you may be able to move it by leaning your back against it and pushing with your legs (wear shoes that grip the floor). If low and stable, it may be possible to move the object by lying on your back on the floor and pushing with your feet.

Ideally, all heavy pieces of furniture should have castors fitted on them to make them easy to move.

Gardening

The same rules apply to gardening jobs as to household ones: lift and carry carefully, using your legs and body weight; work upright whenever practicable; do not do too much at once, and change tasks often; keep the work as close to yourself as possible; get help when necessary.

Avoid prolonged bending and stooping by kneeling down or using a long-handled implement to do the job whenever possible.

For pruning and fruit picking, long-handled implements which allow one to avoid reaching high up above, should be used with care. While they may not be heavy items in themselves, when they are lifted or lowered they put a stress on the back.

Try to keep the sweeps of action in a forward or backward direction, with the minimum of twisting. Avoid any sweeping action across the body: it needs a good deal of work from the muscles of the trunk, and unless they are in working trim, your back may be strained. The secret is foot position, so that every action is a use of balanced body weight. Where space is too cramped, you may do better by getting down on your hands and knees.

Kneeling is a very sensible posture for many jobs in the garden. For a gardener who can neither stoop nor kneel nor squat, raised borders for flowers or a greenhouse with shelves would be possible outlets.

Digging is a traditional back-breaker for those untrained to it. Do not attempt to dig too much at one time. Stand over the job and try not to overload the fork or spade.

The wheelbarrow puts considerable stress on the spine because it has to be lifted and at the same time pushed – all very well if the ground is hard and level, but a great effort when the ground is soft and steep or uneven. If you need to make use of a wheelbarrow, choose one which takes the load well forward over the wheel; then, when you load it, make sure to place the load over the wheel so that the lifting effort needed is small. Be sure to lift the barrow correctly: stand between the shafts, bending at the hips and knees to reach the handles, then straighten at the hips and knees, lean forward with your body weight – and move off. It is better to make two journeys with small loads than to struggle with one.

Mowing the lawn

Lawnmowers are heavy, yet have to be heaved backwards, humped over lawn edges and in and out of sheds. Pushed mowers are the lightest and comparatively easy to manoeuvre. When using a push mower, wear boots or shoes with good grip and use your body weight to help the movements.

Of the powered mowers, the lightest are those with electric motors which run off the mains, followed by those with petrol engines; the heaviest, weighing nearly 100 lb, are electric mowers which run off accumulators. Cylinder mowers are on the whole heavier than rotary mowers, but, being more compact, are easier to manoeuvre. Rotary mowers are handy for rough grass but there the effort of manoeuvring is far greater, particularly if the mower has small wheels.

Many people empty the grass box into a wheelbarrow but unless you have an ergonomically satisfactory barrow or cart, it may be easier to empty the grass box on to a sheet with handles at the corners which is easy to pull across the lawn to the compost tip.

With mowing, as with all gardening and other heavy work, the rule is not to do too much at a time. Plan all the work so that you can divide it into many short sessions, rather than a few long ones, and allow plenty of time to do the work. If working alongside somebody else, do not feel that you have to keep up; work at your own pace. If your back starts hurting, do not struggle on to finish because the weather is right or you are going away tomorrow – stop.

Driving a car

Driving is an activity which gives a lot of people backache, even if they are otherwise free of back trouble. The problem is basically that the driver is working in a flexed posture, and the effects are made much worse by any deficiencies in the design and construction of the seat itself. Most car seats give poor lumbar support, and no lateral thigh support.

Adjust the car seat and angle of the back rest so that the pedals and the gear lever and steering wheel can be comfortably reached. When the driver's knees are bent up too high because the seat will not go back far enough, the remedy may be to have the seat raised on blocks – provided this can be done securely and there is enough headroom. In most cars, the runners of the seat can be moved so that you have more backward and forward positions. Before you make alterations to your driving seat, check that this will not interfere with your vision and control.

First the seat, then the car

Anybody buying a new car should ensure that the seat is adjustable, but should also try and have an opportunity of driving someone else's car of the same make for at least half an hour. If this is not possible, travelling as a front seat passenger in the car may give some idea as to whether the seat of that particular make is suitable for a person with back problems. It is not possible to form a true impression by sitting in a stationary vehicle. When trying out a new car seat, it takes about half an hour of continuous driving to be able to predict how comfortable a car seat will be on a long journey.

A car's seat should never be so springy that you bounce more than it does, and the padding should give lateral support to prevent your being thrown sideways on cornering, otherwise the spine is unsupported. If there is not enough lumbar support, use a cushion or anything that gives support in the small of the back. However, it is better not to use an inflatable cushion: this will aggravate the problem of lack of sideways control, because on cornering and pressing on pedals, air in the cushion may move to the 'wrong' side and this will tend to force the body into an even worse lateral displacement.

Car accessory shops sell numerous aids to seat comfort. Anything that supports your lower back and prevents it from flexing, or gives added sideways support, may help. Wooden bead mats that hang on the back of the seat are found helpful by some people. A back rest can be individually moulded to fit you in any seat, but you must be able to fix it securely to the car seat – ask the supplier about this. Remember, however, that anything inserted for seat comfort occupies space and reduces the effective length of the seat. The Disabled Living Foundation (see p. 100) has up-to-date information about supports that are available.

Driving

Backache from car driving is partly a postural stress but some of it comes from the movements of the car transmitted to the driver.

While driving, you scarcely change your position and your range of movement is restricted by the position of the hand and foot controls. Try to be relaxed while driving. To help prevent tenseness and stiffness in the neck, whenever you have to stop – for instance, at lights or in traffic jams – move the neck about a bit: shrug your shoulders a few times, raising them as high as possible towards your ears and then suddenly drop them.

It helps on a long journey to stop and take a little exercise at frequent intervals. Taking a short walk, even just around the car, provides a change of position, and therefore movement of the back. When stopping for petrol, always get out of the car.

Getting in and out

When climbing out of a car, get used to swivelling your whole body towards the door; then slide your feet onto the ground together, and stand up. Do not twist round to pick up parcels from the back seat.

A four-door car makes life with small children much easier on the back than a two-door car. If you have the latter, get into the rear with the child, and then strap it into its seat.

Luggage in the car

When travelling by car, there is the problem of loading it. Many car boots have a high sill to hump the luggage over, and this imposes a major stress – especially when having to duck under the lid of the boot. If the floor of the boot is lower than the edge of the boot opening, limit the weight of individual bits of luggage so that they can be easily swung up to rest on the sill of the boot, then lowered with one hand while you support yourself with the other hand. Keep the floor of the boot clear of clutter so that the suitcases can easily be pushed into position. Avoid trying to push things sideways. If you can, move your feet so that you pull things into place rather than having to twist your body to heave them about.

Air travel

Airline seats vary in comfort according to the price. Economy-class seats are designed to be particularly mean with elbow and leg room, but on long journeys, even the more expensive seats can leave you feeling stiff. Get up and walk about now and again if your possibly can.

Sleeping in your seat has to be done in one position – leaning back – and that is usually a sure way to a stiff neck. The inadequate little cushions handed out by the airlines on long-distance flights are not much help: placed behind the neck, they keep sliding out. Most airport shops and luggage shops sell U-shaped inflatable cushions which support the neck quite efficiently, and the airline's cushion can go in the small of your back.

Carrying luggage
Pack and unpack a suitcase downstairs to avoid having to lug it down or up the stairs when it is full and heavy.

A shoulder bag, such as an airline carry-on bag, is better than a hand-held bag, provided this does not lead to uneven posture on one side – try putting the strap diagonally across the body rather than over one shoulder. Or carry two evenly loaded bags, one in each hand.

Suitcases and holdalls can be troublesome to someone liable to back pain. The logical solution to carrying luggage is to divide the load into three: in a rucksack over your shoulders, and one small case in each hand.

A suitcase with its own wheels can take much of the lifting out of moving luggage. Make sure that the handle is at a comfortable

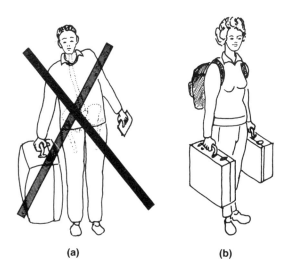

(a)   (b)

(a) Don't carry all your luggage in one big suitcase. The dotted line shows how it affects the spine and pelvis

(b) Better for the spine to spread the load, with a smaller suitcase in each hand and a rucksack on the back

height, that the suitcase comes with a strap to pull it along, otherwise trying to wheel a small suitcase with castors underneath would mean walking with an awkwardly twisted spine.

CHAPTER 16

EXERCISE

IT is a truth universally acknowledged that regular exercise is good for the health. The huge interest in their own health that people in western countries have been showing in recent years has been accompanied by growing participation in many forms of exercise. There are many exercise programmes and schemes to be found, so it is as well to make sure before embarking on any for the first time that they are safe and effective, with properly trained tutors.

Many people who take up sports or games do not follow a regular routine, and risk injuring their health rather than improving it. To be effective and safe, exercise must be regular, and a time of each day should be set aside for it. You should strictly follow a graduated programme of exercises, and as far as possible make sure that you are building up muscular strength on both sides of the vertebral column equally.

Sports and athletics

Each sporting and athletic activity has its own techniques, which must be learned and practised, for preventing damage to joints, ligaments and muscles. Even professional sportsmen, athletes and gymnasts, who train constantly, quite often suffer from strains and sprains, and anybody who goes in for such activities without adequate training and preparation is very likely to suffer for it.

If you go in for sport as relaxation from work, you should be restrained in your ambition, and bring not too competitive a spirit with you which would make you disregard your health and safety.

One golden rule for sport which should always be followed is: warm up before you start. Gymnasts and ballet dancers always start with some gentle exercises designed to warm up joints and muscles which have not been used for a while. They know that to start to work cold is to invite injury. Warm-up exercises should stretch the postural muscles; loosen and stretch all the leg joints and foot joints; stretch the arm and hand joints. If you intend to be involved in sport, it is important to train and play regularly. It is irregular training or playing which is a frequent cause of injury. Do not train or play when you are injured. In attempting to protect one injury you may precipitate another – for example, prolonged limping may aggravate or initiate a back problem.

Which sport?

No sport is good or bad in itself; what counts is how you go about it. But for anyone with back trouble (past or present) some are not advisable such as, obviously, rugby, parachuting, trampolining.

Walking

Both walking and running can be valuable in helping to prevent obesity and are both natural activities which, if done with proper care, make a demand on the postural muscles which may help to prevent back problems. Walking is increasingly the preferred alternative to jogging.

For running or jogging, it is important to reduce the jarring effect which is transmitted to the back if poorly cushioned, badly designed (this usually means cheap) shoes are worn. Old training shoes may also cause trouble because even though the sole is not worn out, the midsole has lost its cushioning powers.

Always wear comfortable, well fitting shoes. Lace-up styles with thick light soles, or trainers are considered ideal. Some people find it useful to add a pair of shock-absorbing insoles or heel pads, obtainable from larger chemists or sports stores.

When walking, walk tall, keep your tummy tucked in and let your arms swing. Start with short walks and gradually increase the distance. As walking becomes easier, increase your speed and stride.

Walking around the shops, dodging people, stopping to look in shop windows and standing at check-outs does not constitute walking as a helpful exercise. In fact, many people who do not otherwise have backache find an afternoon's shopping can cause one. A real walk should be part of your regular routine: around the block or the nearest park to start with and, gradually, as your walking fitness improves, you will be able to go farther afield.

Swimming

Swimming provides the body with good all-round exercise. It encourages mobility and, without putting undue strain on the spine, promotes muscle strength. It is valuable for people with back problems: the water provides support and the exercise can be undertaken without stressing the spinal column. The buoyancy of the water minimises the effects of body weight, making it easier to move.

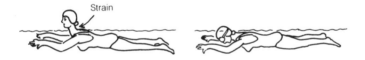

The most effective strokes are the front crawl and the back-stroke which give the whole body regular and rhythmic movement. If you swim breast stroke, try not to keep your head out of the water all the time, as this extended position can put a strain on the neck. Try wearing goggles and learn to breathe out with your face under the water. In this way the head is kept in line with the body and the neck stress minimised.

Exercising at home

Exercises for the back are chiefly intended to strengthen the muscles. The vertebral joints do not need to be exercised, because the spine is never at rest, even when you are in bed. Stiffness in these joints can be helped by exercise only if it is due to weakness in the muscles and ligaments. This can be helped by gently working the muscles. But when there is stiffness as a result of a disc prolapse, misaligned facet joints or curvature, exercises can do harm rather than good.

An important rule is: if an exercise hurts, stop doing it.

Exercises that do not help a bad back

There are some kinds of exercises which should be positively avoided when you are recovering from back pain, and used with caution at all times:

Bending forwards is supposed to strengthen the abdominal muscles, but is not advisable where the pressure can push a disc protrusion into the spinal canal;

Exercises to stretch the spine are given by some instructors to reduce disc protrusion and strengthen back muscles, but excessive extension can damage the facet joints;

Bending sideways can be beneficial in moderation, but always involves some rotation of each vertebra, so that the exercise needs to be done slowly, carefully and over a short range;

Rotation has been thought to mobilise stiff joints, but excessive rotation is harmful: since the immobile joints cannot be moved, the mobile ones will be overstrained;

Toe touching used to be one of the classic exercises for fitness, but to touch your toes while standing (or while sitting) with legs straight and feet apart is likely to do more harm than good, particularly if you use the opposite hand, so adding a twisting motion;

Double leg raising, often recommended as an abdominal strengthening exercise, can be positively harmful because it puts considerable strain on the lower back. During this exercise the hip muscles have to do most work and as they are attached to the lower lumbar vertebrae and the pelvis, the abdominal muscles are called upon to stabilise the pelvis while the legs are lifted. The weight of the straight legs makes it too difficult for the abdominal muscles to continue to hold the pelvis, which tilts forward. This causes the lumbar spine to hollow as the spinal joints are pulled forward, putting considerable strain on them.

Lifting both legs up straight, or **sitting up from lying with a straight back** are two exercises which should not be carried out, except by someone exceptionally fit and well muscled.

Exercises for the back

Movement is necessary for the maintenance of a healthy spine. Regular physical activity helps to ensure that the joints remain mobile and the muscles strong. A stiff spine with weak supporting muscles cannot cope with the additional stress that might be imposed on it by some unaccustomed position or sudden awkward movement.

It is therefore extremely important, if you have a back problem, or have had one in the past, to ensure that your spine is as mobile as possible and supported by strong muscles.

The following exercises, if performed regularly, will help to improve spinal mobility and strengthen the muscles which control the movements and postures of the spine.

Start gently with the easier exercises at the beginning of each section. When you can easily do 12 or 15 repetitions of that exercise, add the next one.

You should not carry out any exercise in a way that causes pain which continues after the exercise is finished. However, if your spine is very stiff, you may feel some discomfort while stretching. As long as this discomfort goes when you stop the exercise, it is likely to be helping to restore your range of movement and will become easier on subsequent occasions. If the discomfort persists, omit that exercise.

Exercises mainly for the lower back

The following exercises are suitable for most people with backache; it has been found that low back pain is more common in people with poor posture, weak abdominal muscles, stiffness and tight hip muscles, especially the psoas and the hamstrings. These exercises, if performed regularly and thoroughly, will help diminish all these pain-causing problems.

To get down on to the floor comfortably, go on to your knees first, then your hands; turn on to one hip and elbow and lower yourself down gently on to your back. To get up, reverse the procedure: on to one hip and elbow, turn on to hands and knees, then one knee, and stand up.

Abdominal strengthening exercises
Start by lying on the floor with knees bent.

1. Rest one hand on your abdomen. Take a deep slow breath in; as you breathe out, gently pull in your abdominal muscles. Repeat 5 times.

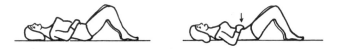

Get into the habit of breathing out when tightening your abdominal muscles: this should help you avoid holding your breath while exercising, which causes an increase in intra-abdominal pressure and thus increases the stress on your spine. You do not have to think about breathing in; it happens automatically.

Practise tightening your abdominal muscles frequently during the day; strong tummy muscles give your back extra protection.

2. Flatten the hollow of your back down on to the floor, at the same time squeeze your buttocks together so that the lower part of your pelvis lifts slightly.

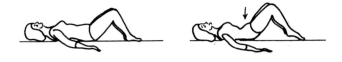

This is a very important exercise which mobilises the lumbar spine, as well as strengthening the abdominal and hip extensor muscles. Practise it in sitting as well as lying, and do it frequently during the day.

3. Lift head and shoulders and slide hands up to knees, keep feet firmly pressed on to the floor. Hold for a count of 4 and lower your head and shoulders.

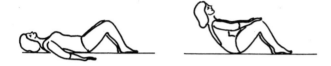

4. Cross arms across chest; lift head and shoulders and reach with the elbow in the direction of the opposite knee; hold for a count of 4. Repeat to the other side.

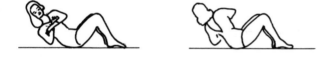

5. Lift both bent knees on to chest: straighten legs towards ceiling; hold; bend knees and put feet back on to floor.
This exercise strengthens the abdominal muscles and stretches the hamstrings.

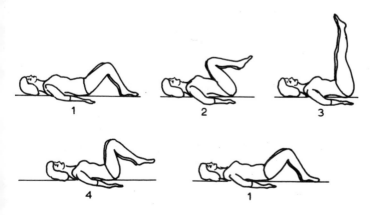

6. Bend knees on to chest: lift buttocks off floor and hold for a count of 4.

This is a very strong abdominal exercise.

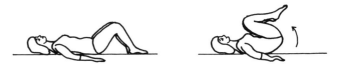

7. Lift both bent knees on to chest. Lift head and shoulders and put hands on knees. Try to push knees away with your hands, at the same time resisting the pressure with your knees.

This is a strong static, or isometric, exercise.

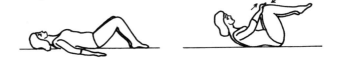

Mobilising and stretching exercises

Start by lying on the floor with knees bent.

1. Keep feet and knees together and let legs drop down from side to side. Progress to doing the same movement with the feet off the floor.

This mobilises the spine and strengthens the abdominal muscles.

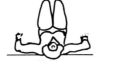

2. Bend one knee on to chest and hold it with both hands; push the straight leg as flat as possible on to the floor. Repeat with the other leg.
This mobilises hips and stretches the psoas muscles.

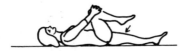

3. From the same position, lift buttocks as high as possible and then lower them. Repeat while raising both arms above head at the same time; next lower yourself on to one hip only, then raise yourself and rotate down on to the other hip.

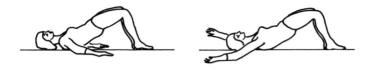

4. Straighten one leg; make the straight leg longer and shorter by tilting the pelvis sideways away from your waist and towards it. Keep the knee straight. Repeat with other leg.

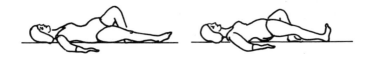

The next two exercises start while you are standing and involve a chair.

5. Stand with your toes about 12 to 18 inches in front of a firm chair. Put one foot up on to the chair and lean forwards. You will feel the stretch in the front of the straight leg. Repeat with the other leg.

This stretches the psoas muscles.

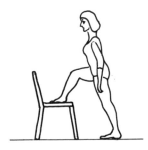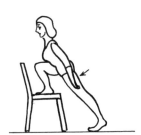

6. This time, put your heel on to the chair and, keeping the knee straight, lean forwards, letting the standing leg bend. Repeat with the other leg.

This stretches the hamstrings.

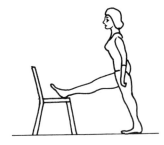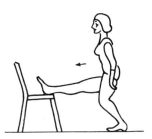

Back and hip extensor strengthening exercises

1. Lie on tummy over a pillow: raise head and shoulders to the horizontal – without arching the back, as this can put a strain on the posterior joints. Progress by repeating with arms stretched sideways.

In this way, the back extensor muscles work, but no stress is put on the joints.

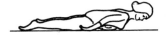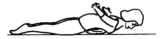

2. Lie trunk over a firm table with a folded towel under hips: hold onto edges of table: lift both legs to horizontal and hold for a count of 4.

This is a very strong extension exercise.

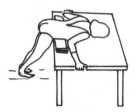
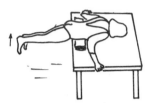

Leg strengthening exercises

Such exercises are important for safe lifting.

1. Sit on a firm chair; hold arms in front; stand up and sit down 10 times. Next stage: sit on a low stool and do the same exercise.

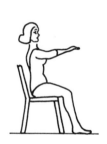
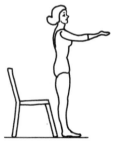
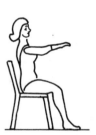

2. As **1**, but on only one leg; repeat with the other leg.

This is a very strong exercise.

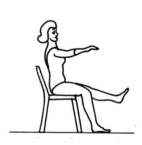
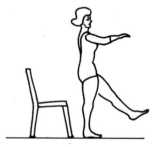

3. Stand on one leg with your eyes closed for a count of 20. Repeat with other leg.

This is an exercise for balance.

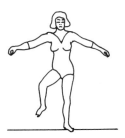 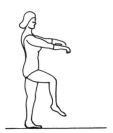

Exercises mainly for the thoracic spine

Women seem particularly vulnerable to thoracic (chest level) spine strain, perhaps from lifting babies in and out of cots and prams, lifting shopping out of the boot of the car, and so on. Try to be aware of the potential problems and straighten the middle part of your back before lifting.

The muscles across the back can feel stretched and ache, pull your shoulder blades together to tighten them.

1. Sit on a chair with knees apart. Bend sideways to reach with one hand down towards the floor; at the same time raise the other arm sideways and backwards, rotating the spine to look at the upstretched arm.

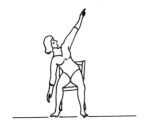

2. Kneel down and sit on heels: bend forwards and rest forehead on floor in front of knees, arms by your side with palms downwards. Keep sitting on heels with ribs touching thighs; lift head and shoulders without arching the neck. Lift arms and turn them so that the back of the hands are facing each other.

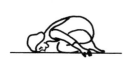 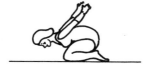

Exercises mainly for the cervical spine

The neck is a common site of spinal pain, but it is an area which responds well to judicious exercise. The posture of the head (which weighs about 12 lbs) is crucial. Try to make the back of the neck so long so that the head is positioned above the shoulders and not in front of them. Experiment by trying to balance a book on your head; this will give you the feeling of good neck posture. Avoid complete head circling movements and extreme extension, as these are unnecessarily stressful to the vertebral joints, and can make you feel dizzy.

The neck and shoulders are often the site for tension pains; try shrugging your shoulders up to your ears several times, this often helps.

1. Lie on back with head on 2 pillows and hips and knees bent; raise head smoothly and press chin on to chest; feel the stretch in the back of the neck; lower gently and repeat 4 times.

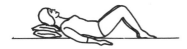 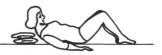

2. Remove one pillow, still keep hips and knees bent, gently turn head to one side, feel the stretch, hold and then turn to the other side. Repeat 4 times.

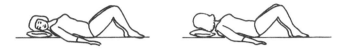

3. Sit on a chair; bend head forwards and gently turn it from side to side: be careful not to arch your head backwards.

4. Stand with head in a good position; take arms in large vigorous circles backwards 10 times and forwards 10 times.

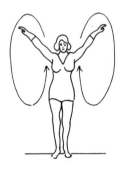

Glossary

Adhesions   Growing-together of tissue due to inflammation

Ankylosing spondylitis   An inflammatory disease of unknown origin, which may affect the mobility of the spine

Annulus fibrosus   Outer casing of intervertebral disc

Apophyseal joint   Facet joint

Arachnoiditis   An inflammation of the arachnoid mater membrane, causing it to thicken, and so impede the movement of nerve roots inside the dural sleeves

Arachnoid mater   See *dural tube*

Arthritis   Inflammation of the joints

Atlas *and* **axis**   The first two cervical vertebrae: the atlas supports the head and, in turn, is supported by the axis; together they permit nodding, side flexion and rotation of the head

Cauda equina   The bundle of lumbar and sacral nerve roots at the end of the spinal cord (Latin – horse's tail)

Cervical   Relating to the neck (Latin – cervix)

Chronic   Of long duration

Coccyx   Termination of the base of the spine; a vestigial tail, consisting of four tiny fused vertebrae

Disc, intervertebral disc   One of the 23 shock-absorbing pads lying between adjacent pairs of vertebral bodies; each consists of a tough, fibrous outer casing (the annulus fibrosus) enclosing a gel-like core (the nucleus pulposus)

Dislocation   Condition of a joint in which the bones become disconnected from each other

Dorsal   An alternative name for the thoracic part of the spine (Latin – dorsum, the back)

Dural sleeves   The sheaths protecting the nerve roots as they branch off from the spinal cord

Dural tube   The sheath of the spinal cord; it consists of three membranes: the innermost one is the pia mater; this is enclosed in the arachnoid mater; the toughest outermost one is the dura mater

Dura mater   See *dural tube*

Epidural root fibrosis   Abnormal increase of fibrous tissue round a nerve root, resulting from inflammation of the dural sleeve

Extensor   Muscle that extends or straightens out a part of the body

Facet joint   Also known as apophyseal joint. The joint formed by the faceted surfaces of the bones which are covered with cartilage and slide over each other inside a fibrous capsule lined with synovial membrane and lubricated with synovial fluid. This type of joint is found between the processes of adjacent vertebrae, and is similar to plane joints in other parts of the body

Fascia   Thin sheet of connective tissue covering a muscle

Fibrin   Protein which forms when blood clots when tissues are injured; it is the body's natural repair material. Adhesions form when the excess fibrin from an injured membrane fastens it to another tissue

Fibrositis   Inflammation of connective tissue fibres: term is used to denote intermittent localised pain in small areas of muscles or ligaments, possibly resulting from tension or bad posture

Foramen (*plural:* **foramina**)   Gap between the pedicles of adjacent vertebrae, through which the nerve roots emerge as they branch out from the spinal cord

Kyphosis   Convex curvature of the spine, which occurs naturally in the thoracic spine and in the region where the sacrum joins the coccyx; if it is excessive, or is present elsewhere in the spine, it is a deformity. See also *lordosis*

Lamina (*plural:* **laminae**)   A part of the neural arch, lying between the spinous process and the pedicle

Lesion Any unfavourable change in the functioning or texture of organs and tissues; used by some doctors to mean a change assumed to be the cause of pain

Ligament Band of fibrous tissue binding the bones of a joint; it controls the range of movement by allowing it only in certain directions

Lordosis A concave curvature of the spine, which occurs naturally in the cervical and the lumbar spine; if it is excessive or occurs elsewhere in the spine, it is a deformity.
See also *kyphosis*

Lumbago Imprecise term meaning pain in the lumbar region: low back pain

Lumbar Relating to the area of the back between the thoracic spine and the sacrum (Latin – lumbum, the loin)

Myelography X-ray visualisation (using radio-opaque dye) of the space inside the spinal canal surrounding the spinal cord and nerve roots

Nerve root The origin of a nerve as it leaves the spinal cord; one of a pair of bands of nervous tissue branching out of the spinal cord at the level of each vertebra, and passing outwards through a foramen

Neural arch The ring of bone at the back of each vertebra; it is made up of the following projections: two pedicles, two transverse processes, two superior and two inferior articular processes and the spinous process

Nucleus pulposus The gel-like core of an intervertebral disc

Osteoarthritis See *osteoarthrosis*

Osteoarthrosis Degeneration of joints, generally accompanied by the thickening of bone; also called osteoarthritis, but it is not an inflammatory condition

Osteomalacia Bone disease in which vitamin D deficiency in adults causes loss of calcium from, and softening of, the bones

Osteophyte Bony outgrowth or spur forming on a bone or in fibrous tissues attached to a bone

Osteophytosis The proliferation of osteophytes at more than one site, usually accompanied by general thickening of bone

Osteoporosis Bone disease characterised by loss of bone substance, thus making bones more easily fractured

Paget's disease Bone disease in which bones become thicker, but also softer, tending to deform

Pedicle Part of the neural arch; each neural arch has two pedicles

Pia mater See *dural tube*

Processes Bony projections forming part of the neural arch

Prolapse In the case of an intervertebral disc, this means the rupture of the disc's outer casing, and the leaking out of part of the nucleus through the rupture

Reflex Involuntary reaction of the muscles to some stimulus which does not rise to the level of consciousness; reflex actions such as jerking the hand away when touching a hot object, are controlled by the nerves of the spinal cord

Retrolisthesis A backwards displacement of one or more vertebrae

Rheumatism Not a disease, but a vague term used for aches and pains in muscles and joints

Rheumatoid arthritis Inflammatory disease, which may be progressive, of the synovial joints in any part of the body

Sacroiliac joint Joint occurring between each side of the sacrum and the adjoining part of the pelvis called the ilium

Sacrum Curved, wedge-shaped bone, consisting of five fused vertebrae, at the lower end of the spine, between the two halves of the pelvis

Sciatica Not a disease, but the name given to a sharp pain in the area of distribution of the sciatic nerve – that is, along the back of the thigh and down the whole leg; sciatic pain can arise when a disorder of the lumbar spine causes pressure on a nerve root

Scoliosis A sideways curvature of the spine. A structural scoliosis may be a congenital deformity; a postural scoliosis occurs when the spine is bent to reduce pressure on a compressed nerve root and so lessen the pain

Slipped disc A misnomer for a prolapsed disc; intervertebral discs do not slip

Spasm; muscular spasm An involuntary muscular response to injury; the muscles automatically tighten round the site, and this serves to prevent movement of the painful tissues; spasm occurs as a result of over-excitation or stimulation of muscle cells by nerve impulses

Spinal canal The conduit formed by the neural arches and bodies of the vertebrae through which the spinal cord passes

Spinal cord A continuation of the brain along the spinal canal, in the form of a long band of nervous tissue, inside the dural tube; it is the main highway of the nervous system, conveying information to and from the brain

Spondylitis Inflammation of vertebrae

Spondylolisthesis A deformity of the spine in which a vertebra slips forward on the one below, so that the whole of the spine above it is also displaced

Spondylolysis Fracture of the neural arch which may be the cause of spondylolisthesis

Spondylosis Osteoarthritis of the facet joints together with degeneration of discs; the bone thickening may result in encroachment into the spinal canal

Stenosis Narrowing of some passage or canal in the body. Lateral stenosis occurs when for some reason the width of a foramen is restricted, compressing the nerve root inside it; central canal stenosis occurs when the spinal cord is compressed by some reduction in the width of the spinal canal

Subluxation When the bones in a joint are displaced but not completely dislocated

Synovial joint Joint enclosed in a fibrous capsule lined with the synovial membrane

Synovium (synovial membrane) Moist membrane lining the capsule which encloses a synovial joint (for example a facet joint); it is lubricated with synovial fluid

Tendon Tough fibrous elongation of a muscle, serving to attach it to a bone

Thoracic Relating to the chest (Latin – thorax)

Vertebra (*plural* **vertebrae)**   One of the 24 bones, stacked on top of each other and separated by discs, which, together with the sacrum and the coccyx, make up the spinal column. Each vertebra (except for the atlas and the axis) consists of a solid body, out of which extends the neural arch

INDEX

(gl refers to glossary)

OTHER PUBLICATIONS FROM WHICH?

Understanding Headaches and Migraines £8. 95

This practical book looks at the various factors which can cause or contribute to headaches and sorts out the everyday and easily manageable headaches from migraines and other more serious types of headache which require further action. Written by one of Britain's most distinguished neurologists, Dr J N Blau, this book offers guidance and support on how to cope, and advises when you ought to see a doctor and what to expect if you are referred to a specialist or directed to a particular type of treatment. In addition, the book looks at complementary therapies and contains a list of migraine clinics in the United Kingdom.

Understanding Stress £7. 95

Stress is inherent in the human condition and our century has intensified many stresses and added new ones, many of them psychological or social in nature. Some stresses are related to, or follow on, a specific identifiable event in the person's life: death, divorce, imprisonment rank high on the list. This book deals with stress and life events, stress from the world around us, at work, in the family. It explains the bodily reactions to stress, how to recognise the warning signs and how to help oneself cope with stress.

Healthy Eating – Fact and Fiction £7.95

Healthy Eating – Fact and Fiction is a guide to the long-term implications of diet. It examines the evidence that various diseases and illnesses are linked to our intake of certain foods and offers practical ways of improving your eating habits for the better – without resorting to drastic action. A unique question-naire, specially devised in conjunction with the Nuffield Labora-tories of Comparative Medicine in London, is included to help you assess how much saturated fat, salt, sugar and fibre you actually eat.

Getting Work Done on Your House £7.95

This book explains in straightforward terms the procedure for getting building work done. It deals with the situation of using a professional as a designer and co-ordinator, and with the more vulnerable situation of going it alone and employing a builder on your own. It has been written for the ordinary home owner who has no particular knowledge or experience of the building industry. The book covers both small and more substantial building projects as well as emergency repair work. It does not tell you what sort of repair to carry out or what type of improvement will be most suitable. But, once you have decided what to do, it tells you how to get someone to carry out the work on your behalf.

What to do When Someone Dies £8.95

This companion volume to *Wills and Probate* aims to help those who have never had to deal with the arrangements that must be made after a death – getting a doctor's certificate and registering the death, deciding whether to bury or cremate, choosing an undertaker and a coffin, putting notices in the papers, selecting the form of service, claiming national insurance benefits. It explains the function of people with whom the bereaved will come in contact, often for the first time. They will get help and guidance from the doctor, the registrar, the undertaker, the clergyman, the cemetery or crematorium officials, the Department of Social Security and, in some circumstances, the police and the coroner. However, it is the executor or nearest relative who has to make the decisions, often at a time of personal distress. The book describes what needs to be done, when, and how to set about it. No attempt is made to deal with the personal or social aspects of death, such as the psychology of grief and shock, the rituals and conventions of mourning, or attitudes to death.

Wills and Probate   £8.95

There are still too many people who have not made their will. This book will help them to do so, not blindly but aware of all the tax implications, the consequences of divorce, the right choice of executors, the proper signing and witnessing of the will so that their wishes can be carried out simply and sensibly. The second part of the book describes what has to be done, administratively, by the executors of the estate of someone who has died. The probate registry provides special machinery to deal with laymen who wish to do so without dealing with a solicitor. *Wills and Probate* supplements this by explaining, in detail, not only the probate registry procedure but all that goes before and what comes after. It also highlights recent relevant changes in tax law and procedure.

This book explains the law and procedure in England and Wales and briefly explains the main differences which apply in Scotland.

Starting Your Own Business   £8.95

It's in at the deep end for many people who want to set up their own business. It represents a challenge and an adventure, but needs hard information on finance, marketing, tax, insurance, premises, employing others and, above all, how to choose the right business project.

Starting Your Own Business explains the steps to be taken for the getting and the spending of business money, from applying for a government grant and taking advantage of agencies that offer funds and advice, to cash flow forecasting, pricing policy, keeping business records and preparing a balance sheet. It discusses the different ways of trading, the pros and cons of franchises or buying an existing business, and explains the law for consumers – from the other side of the counter.

This book was first published in 1983 – since then, everyone in Britain has become aware of the part that small businesses have to play in the economy. Whatever business the reader is thinking of starting, there is a lot to be learned and a lot of information to be gathered.

Earning Money at Home £8.95

This popular book explains how to brush up a skill or hobby into a money-making venture. It gives advice on organising your family and domestic life, on advertising your activities, costing and selling your work, dealing with customers. There is information on statutory and financial requirements for insurance, tax, accounts, VAT, employing others. The book suggests ways in which your experience from a previous job could be utilised, or a skill or hobby developed to a professional standard, or how unexploited energy and ability can be used profitably. Suggestions are made for improving your skills, and the names and addresses are given of organisations that might be helpful.

The Which? Guide to Planning and Conservation £8.95

This helpful guide sets out the circumstances in which householders need planning permission and describes the special rules that apply to listed buildings and conservation areas. This book offers advice on how to go about getting planning permission and how to appeal if permission is withheld, as well as explaining what rights householders have to help protect their homes against neighbours' plans. It also includes a section on campaigning against major developments in order to help conserve your environment.

You and the Environment   £8.95

You and the Environment addresses the question of what the individual can do to reduce the damage being done to the environment, not only by relating global problems to the individual consumer but by demonstrating what we can do to become more environmentally friendly. As well as looking at the pros and cons of recycling schemes, at the benefits of using less water in the house and at the advantages of organic food, the book offers advice about such matters as saving energy and reducing waste. Full of practical tips, it describes what every one of us can do to take responsibility for the world in which we live.

Which Subject? Which Career?   £8.95

This new edition of *Which Subject? Which Career?* has been fully revised and updated to take account of the major changes in the world of education, including the implementation of the National Curriculum. It considers the choices facing teenagers at 14, when they currently select their GCSE subjects; at 16, when they sit GCSE or leave school for a job, vocational training or further education, and at 18, with A-levels, jobs or higher education. It also describes higher education for the 18-plus age-group and has a new chapter on sponsorship and grants.

This is an invaluable handbook which gives details of over 200 careers, from accountancy to zoology, and explains the qualifications needed for them.

You and Your Pension   £7.95

You and Your Pension takes an in-depth look at the methods you can choose for retirement saving – whatever your circumstances. Whether you are years away from retirement and have time to plan ahead, are looking for a way to boost an existing pension or simply want to know the steps for claiming pensions, this book offers all the information and advice you need to help you make the right choices. It also includes a number of useful examples, tables and charts to aid your understanding.

Divorce – Legal Procedures and Financial Facts £7.95

This guide explains the special procedure for an undefended divorce and deals with the financial facts to be faced when a marriage ends in divorce. Aspects covered include getting legal advice, conciliation, legal aid and its drawbacks, the various financial and property orders the court can make, what can happen to the matrimonial home, the children, how to calculate needs and resources, the effect of tax, coping with shortage of money after divorce.

Which? also produces a number of handy **Action Packs** which offer information, advice and practical aids, such as loose-leaf worksheets, forms and directories, all in one neat package. Titles include *Buying a Second-hand Car, How to Sort out Someone's Will* and *Baby on the Way*. These and other *Which?* publications are available from the *Which?* shop at 359/361 Euston Road, London NW1 3AL, or by post (no charge for post and packing) from Consumers' Association, Castlemead, Gascoyne Way, Hertford X, SG14 1LH and from booksellers